HEALTH CARE IN TRANSITION

PHARMACISTS

CURRENT CHALLENGES AND PERSPECTIVES

HEALTH CARE IN TRANSITION

Additional books and e-books in this series can be found on Nova's website under the Series tab.

HEALTH CARE IN TRANSITION

PHARMACISTS

CURRENT CHALLENGES AND PERSPECTIVES

LINE L. VILLADSEN
EDITOR

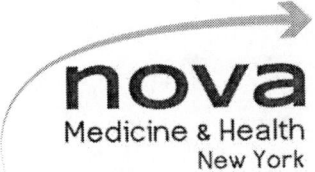

Copyright © 2020 by Nova Science Publishers, Inc.

All rights reserved. No part of this book may be reproduced, stored in a retrieval system or transmitted in any form or by any means: electronic, electrostatic, magnetic, tape, mechanical photocopying, recording or otherwise without the written permission of the Publisher.

We have partnered with Copyright Clearance Center to make it easy for you to obtain permissions to reuse content from this publication. Simply navigate to this publication's page on Nova's website and locate the "Get Permission" button below the title description. This button is linked directly to the title's permission page on copyright.com. Alternatively, you can visit copyright.com and search by title, ISBN, or ISSN.

For further questions about using the service on copyright.com, please contact:
Copyright Clearance Center
Phone: +1-(978) 750-8400   Fax: +1-(978) 750-4470   E-mail: info@copyright.com.

NOTICE TO THE READER

The Publisher has taken reasonable care in the preparation of this book, but makes no expressed or implied warranty of any kind and assumes no responsibility for any errors or omissions. No liability is assumed for incidental or consequential damages in connection with or arising out of information contained in this book. The Publisher shall not be liable for any special, consequential, or exemplary damages resulting, in whole or in part, from the readers' use of, or reliance upon, this material. Any parts of this book based on government reports are so indicated and copyright is claimed for those parts to the extent applicable to compilations of such works.

Independent verification should be sought for any data, advice or recommendations contained in this book. In addition, no responsibility is assumed by the Publisher for any injury and/or damage to persons or property arising from any methods, products, instructions, ideas or otherwise contained in this publication.

This publication is designed to provide accurate and authoritative information with regard to the subject matter covered herein. It is sold with the clear understanding that the Publisher is not engaged in rendering legal or any other professional services. If legal or any other expert assistance is required, the services of a competent person should be sought. FROM A DECLARATION OF PARTICIPANTS JOINTLY ADOPTED BY A COMMITTEE OF THE AMERICAN BAR ASSOCIATION AND A COMMITTEE OF PUBLISHERS.

Additional color graphics may be available in the e-book version of this book.

Library of Congress Cataloging-in-Publication Data

Names: Villadsen, Line L., editor.
Title: Pharmacists : current challenges and perspectives / Line L.
   Villadsen, editor.
Description: New York : Nova Science Publishers, [2020] | Series: Health
   care in transition | Includes bibliographical references and index. |
Identifiers: LCCN 2020020542 (print) | LCCN 2020020543 (ebook) | ISBN
   9781536180183 (paperback) | ISBN 9781536180190 (adobe pdf)
Subjects: LCSH: Pharmacy. | Pharmacists--Training of. | Pharmacy--Study and
   teaching.
Classification: LCC RS122.5 .P4724 2020 (print) | LCC RS122.5 (ebook) |
   DDC 615.1--dc23
LC record available at https://lccn.loc.gov/2020020542
LC ebook record available at https://lccn.loc.gov/2020020543

Published by Nova Science Publishers, Inc. † New York

CONTENTS

Preface		vii
Chapter 1	Addressing the Gap between Pharmacy Education and Practice *Nilay Aksoy*	1
Chapter 2	Current Challenges and Perspectives of Pharmacist in Oncology Settings *Songül Tezcan*	39
Chapter 3	Current Challenges and Perspectives of Pharmacy in Middle Eastern Countries *Hala Sacre, Souheil Hallit, Aline Hajj and Pascale Salameh*	69
Chapter 4	Pharmacists in Low- and Middle-Income Countries: Challenges and Perspectives *Thang Nguyen, Linh T. K. Mai, Vu T. Nguyen, Thu T. A. Truong, Tu T. C. Le, Suol T. Pham, Chu X. Duong, Thao H. Nguyen, Susan E. Matthews and Katja Taxis*	129

Chapter 5	Synthesis of Relevant Information to Support Multi-Criteria Decision Analysis (MCDA) for Pharmacist Decision-Making *Alberto Frutos Pérez-Surio*	**163**
Index		**187**

PREFACE

It has become apparent that pharmacy education needs to respond to professional and social changes and renew its mission in terms of students and learning objectives. As such, this compilation presents approaches for bridging the theory-practice gap. Following this, the authors focus on pharmacists' role in oncology, and the current challenges and perspectives of pharmacist in oncology settings. Oncology pharmacists contribute to the rational use of chemotherapy and supportive drugs by providing individual pharmaceutical care plans for patients. Challenges in pharmacy education and practice in the Middle East are discussed, and the authors elaborate on specific frameworks for different sectors of pharmacy. It is also proposed that developing the pharmacist's role as a major part of the medical team could provide patients with the highest outcomes at the lowest cost. The objective of the closing review is to make a proposal for the implementation of the analysis of ethical, organisational, legal, social, environmental and other domains, in the studies of the health technology assessment agencies. (Imprint: Nova Medicine and Health)

Chapter 1 - The heath care process is struggling with complexity, yielding the necessity for multidisciplinary approaches involving all health care providers as well as social scientists and well-rounded pharmacists. The discrepancy between training and practice makes it difficult to undertake these approaches. It has become apparent that pharmacy education needs to respond to professional and social changes and renew its mission in terms of students and learning objectives. "In theory, there is no difference between theory and practice, but in practice there is," stated Manfred Eigen. This chapter will focus on approaches for bridging the theory-practice gap.

First of all, these differences can be resolved by carrying out realistic research. Pharmacy institutions should perform advanced research to determine the needs and to promote and support the practice. Numerous literature studies support the proposition to include pharmacists in inter-professional primary health care teams. Country-based research will help confirm whether the training system and education obtained by pharmacy students is sufficient to promote a positive attitude toward potential integration into primary health care.

Second, common, clear, and compelling outcomes should be established based on previous studies, and education should be standardized accordingly. A well-rounded student of pharmacy is created by a high-quality pharmacy school, a well-formed curriculum that meets the requirements, and a highly effective style and method of education. The curriculum of apprenticeships should be improved. The enhancement of apprenticeship programs should not be limited to increasing the number of apprenticeship courses, but should also extend to the quality of their content. Simulation training can play an important role in upscaling and improving pharmacy learning productivity and in overcoming the barrier of limited real-field learning.

Lastly, the disparity between community-based and hospital-based apprenticeships and the courses attributed to graduates must be reduced to provide compatibility with pharmacy practice. Inter-professional education (IPE) should be introduced into the curriculum. One of the major obstacles to the success of the pharmacist in providing primary health care is presented when the pharmacist is directly involved in patient care and this role is ignored by other health care providers. Inter-professional education prepares students for collaborative thinking and practice. Building this collaborative project through education has a major impact on bridging the gaps between different providers of primary health care.

Preface

In summary, the recommendations proposed include: continuing professional development (CPD) to enhance the workforce, incorporating technologies and software in pharmacy education, evaluating the education process from different aspects (students, practitioners, primary health care providers), restructuring the curriculum according to research feedback, and finally, effectively collaborating with other health care providers ("One hand can't clap alone").

Chapter 2 - Multidisciplinary approach is one of the corner stones of the successful cancer therapy. Pharmacist as a health advisor in multidisciplinary team has a vital role in oncology setting. The oncology pharmacists (OPs) are the specialist pharmacists on oncology and involved in the planning and administration of chemotherapy, which is the most common cancer treatment. OPs in the multidisciplinary team contribute to the rational use of chemotherapy and supportive drugs by providing individual pharmaceutical care plans for patients. Pharmaceutical care is a new discipline, which was first defined, by Charles D. Hepler and Linda M. Strand in 1990. The definition of pharmaceutical care has been improved with some changes over time. According to these definitions; the pharmacist's responsibilities include preventing, identifying and solving the drug related problems (DRPs), providing patient-oriented service, making a care plan, following up patients. Recent studies have shown that pharmaceutical care programs have positive contributions to the treatment of oncology patients. The increasing incidence of cancer cases and the development of new drugs lead to application of personalized therapies. Many studies have shown that OPs contribute to optimize the medication use and to provide rationale therapy. However, during pharmaceutical care process, OPs sometimes face to challenges with doctors, patients, nurses and other health professionals. This chapter will focus on pharmacist role in oncology and current challenges and perspectives of pharmacist in oncology settings.

Chapter 3 - Introduction: The pharmacy profession in the Middle East is facing several challenges with common features related to the system, education, and practice, as the vast majority of the population live in low- to middle-income countries.

Challenges: From an educational point of view, pharmacy suffers from several gaps: the use of classical teaching methods making little use of digital and active learning methods, the graduation of non-specialized pharmacists with a rare recognition of specialties, the non-application of quality standards in all institutions despite the presence of regional standards, and the dearth of research in pharmaceutical sciences. An additional major issue is the lack of coordination between pharmacy educational institutions and market labor stakeholders, leading to a mismatch between the learning outcomes, competencies and skills of new graduate pharmacists, and continuing professional development programs. Practice challenges consist mainly in shifting the perceived image of the pharmacist from a drug seller to a medication expert, by adopting the pharmacist's modern and internationally recognized roles ("The Nine-Star Pharmacist") and by including the clinical, ethical and research aspects of the profession in everyday practice. There is an oversupply of pharmacists in some countries, while other countries suffer from a deep need. The misdistribution of interprofessional tasks, the financial and administrative difficulties associated with the system, and the increased societal demand add to the complexity of pharmaceutical services offered by pharmacists in different sectors.

Perspectives: To overcome these challenges, pharmacists' associations in collaboration with stakeholders in the region, must develop appropriate strategic plans; it is also necessary that governmental and educational institutions recognize and consider specialized competencies and degrees, adopt and implement good pharmacy practice quality standards in community and hospital settings, and apply governance principles. The elaboration of core and specific competencies frameworks for different sectors of pharmacy would help bridging the gap between education and practice. Interprofessional education, collaboration, and communication are additional concepts to be applied in appropriate settings.

Chapter 4 - Over the last decades, there have been several changes in the pharmacist's role in the primary care system due to the establishment of clinical pharmacy and community pharmacy. Their contribution to the translation of evidence-based knowledge into clinical practice is helpful in the optimisation of the use of drugs. For example, pharmacists provide recommendations to both medical staff and society in the treatment and prevention of diseases. They are not only responsible for preventing medication errors and solving drug-problems but also providing pharmaceutical care services, especially in chronic disorders. However, in low- and middle- income countries, this clinical practice is a very new area and pharmacists face many social barriers to improve their role. The awareness of the community about the pharmacist's role is still limited and there are many conflicts between pharmacists and other medical staff. Lack of human resources and investments are also challenging for developing the role of clinical and community pharmacists. Raising the knowledge of citizens and developing a way to cope with these barriers is essential to developing the pharmacists' roles as a major part of the medical team and provide patients with the highest outcomes and lowest cost.

Chapter 5 - Introduction Decision-making in healthcare is often complex and involves consideration of numerous factors, hence many of these processes require careful assessment of existing health technologies, as well as the consideration of multiple dimensions to analyze the value of available options. Currently, some countries support macro and meso decision-making in the field of health on economic concepts, with the budgetary impact of the technologies being a major criterion. Further, the Anglo-Saxon model based on cost-utility analysis is used, which provides an estimate that relates the Quality Adjusted Life Years (QALYs) with the costs of health technology. Such analysis is widely used by health technology assessment (HTA) agencies, academia, as well as in industry.

However, value and its dimensions are more complex if we seek to make decisions based on the value of medications. The use of structured and explicit approaches that require the evaluation of multiple criteria containing value dimensions can significantly improve the quality of pharmacy decision-making. Multi-criteria decision analysis (MCDA) is a complementary decision-making tool that can systematically incorporate, in addition to the costs and benefits of medical innovations, other dimensions such as ethical, organisational, legal, environmental and social aspects, together with the perspectives of the various stakeholders.

Aims and Objectives The objective of this review is to make a proposal for the implementation of the analysis of ethical, organisational, legal, social, environmental and other domains, in the studies of the HTA agencies, enabling the incorporation of well-informed MCDA approaches into pharmacist decision-making.

Methods: In order to know the scientific evidence on MCDA techniques in which non-core criteria were used or included for decision-making on the incorporation, modification or exclusion of health technologies, a systematic review was carried out using structured searches in biomedical databases and webpages of different HTA organisations, to sum up the criteria that should be part of each of the aforementioned non-core domains.

Results: As a result of the search for scientific evidence, 42 articles were included that used non-core criteria for the evaluation of health technologies. A total of 216 non-core criteria were extracted and classified by the researchers from these articles, of which 56 were included in the social (socioeconomic) domain, 59 in the organizational, 10 in the legal, 8 in the environmental, 47 in the ethical and 36 in other domains. Of the 216 non-core criteria obtained from the systematic review, 26 criteria were necessary for pharmacist decision-making. These criteria were grouped by domain as follows: five criteria for each of the ethical, legal and environmental domains, four for the social domain and the other domain, and three for the organizational domain.

Conclusion: The 26 selected criteria should be considered by HTA agencies when collecting and synthesizing information for pharmacist decision-making. The consensus group does not consider that some of the domains should be weighed above others or that some individual criteria are more preeminent than others. It is proposed to use MCDA models within a deliberative process and to include it in the information to be retrieved in the process of evaluation of health technologies. These models can serve as a frame of reference in a systematic and structured discussion based on individual criteria and the evidence supporting them. Structured and informed deliberative models have a certain advantage over closed and uninformed decision-making processes, as they make explicit and transparent the reasoning behind the final decision.

In: Pharmacists
Editor: Line L. Villadsen

ISBN: 978-1-53618-018-3
© 2020 Nova Science Publishers, Inc.

Chapter 1

ADDRESSING THE GAP BETWEEN PHARMACY EDUCATION AND PRACTICE

Nilay Aksoy[*]
Clinical Pharmacy, Altinbas University, Istanbul, Turkey

ABSTRACT

The heath care process is struggling with complexity, yielding the necessity for multidisciplinary approaches involving all health care providers as well as social scientists and well-rounded pharmacists. The discrepancy between training and practice makes it difficult to undertake these approaches.

It has become apparent that pharmacy education needs to respond to professional and social changes and renew its mission in terms of students and learning objectives. "In theory, there is no difference between theory and practice, but in practice there is," stated Manfred Eigen. This chapter will focus on approaches for bridging the theory-practice gap.

First of all, these differences can be resolved by carrying out realistic research. Pharmacy institutions should perform advanced research to determine the needs and to promote and support the practice. Numerous literature studies support the proposition to include pharmacists in inter-

---

[*] Corresponding Author's Email: nilay.aksoy@altinbas.edu.tr.

professional primary health care teams. Country-based research will help confirm whether the training system and education obtained by pharmacy students is sufficient to promote a positive attitude toward potential integration into primary health care.

Second, common, clear, and compelling outcomes should be established based on previous studies, and education should be standardized accordingly. A well-rounded student of pharmacy is created by a high-quality pharmacy school, a well-formed curriculum that meets the requirements, and a highly effective style and method of education. The curriculum of apprenticeships should be improved. The enhancement of apprenticeship programs should not be limited to increasing the number of apprenticeship courses, but should also extend to the quality of their content. Simulation training can play an important role in upscaling and improving pharmacy learning productivity and in overcoming the barrier of limited real-field learning.

Lastly, the disparity between community-based and hospital-based apprenticeships and the courses attributed to graduates must be reduced to provide compatibility with pharmacy practice. Inter-professional education (IPE) should be introduced into the curriculum. One of the major obstacles to the success of the pharmacist in providing primary health care is presented when the pharmacist is directly involved in patient care and this role is ignored by other health care providers. Inter-professional education prepares students for collaborative thinking and practice. Building this collaborative project through education has a major impact on bridging the gaps between different providers of primary health care.

In summary, the recommendations proposed include: continuing professional development (CPD) to enhance the workforce, incorporating technologies and software in pharmacy education, evaluating the education process from different aspects (students, practitioners, primary health care providers), restructuring the curriculum according to research feedback, and finally, effectively collaborating with other health care providers ("One hand can't clap alone").

Keywords: pharmacy education, practice, curriculum, simulation, Interprofessional education, technologies

1. THE PRACTICE OF PHARMACY

1.1. History of Pharmacy as a Profession

Pharmacy is an ancient profession, demonstrated by evidence from ancient Sumerian cuneiform and Egyptian papyrus documents recording medicinal prescriptions (Borchardt 2002). Although Hippocrates is considered the founder of medicine, in Ancient Greece before, during, and after the time of Hippocrates, there existed a group of experts in medicinal plants (Kremers et al. 1986). Galen (130–200 A.D.) introduced the preparation and compounding of medicines that were used in the Western world for 1,500 years, and his name is still identified with that class of compounded pharmaceuticals called *galenicals*. Indian, Ephesian, Japanese, and Egyptian histories include several details that emphasize medicinal drug use, as well as job descriptions similar to those of modern pharmacists (Titsimgh 1834).

Historically, there had been no distinction in Europe between the duties of the doctor and the duties of the herbalists until 1683, when the Bruges City Council forbade doctors to prepare medicines for their patients.

The use of herbal medicines had been entirely based on empiricism up to the 18th century. After World War II, the growth of the pharmaceutical industry led to the discovery and use of new and effective drug substances. The function of the pharmacist also changed. The post-war period from the 1950s to the 1990s saw significant advances in drug development with the introduction of new antibiotics and analgesics and the creation of new medication groups (Taylor 2015). Over the years, pharmacy has grown from a traditional and generic drug-based profession to one with an advanced, patient-focused basis (Toklu and Hussain 2013).

1.2. Changing Aspects

Pharmacists were more engaged in the compounding and manufacturing of medicines in the past century, but over time, this function has diminished considerably. This progress in the practice enables pharmacists to be part of the multidisciplinary health care team working to provide patients with better healthcare, and thereby contributing to the achievement of global goals (Toklu and Hussain 2013).

1.3. Functional Models

Numerous functional models have been developed for pharmacy including the models of (1) drug information practice, (2) self-care practice, (3) clinical pharmacy practice, (4) pharmaceutical care, (5) medication therapy management, and (6) distributive practice (Wiedenmayer et al. 2006).

1.3.1. Drug Information Model

The pharmacy and pharmacotherapy fields are areas of rapid change, with continuous introduction of new approaches, new products, and new information about old products.

Evidence-based medicine (EBM) or pharmacy tries to move the practice away from a circumstantial and empirical approach and to rely on the best possible evidence for the success of a medicine or procedure. Pharmacists should be knowledgeable in EBM so they can respond appropriately to clinical questions. Application of EBM also enables the pharmacist to carefully analyze physician instructions and to find more suitable and pharmaco-economic alternative medications (Wiedenmayer et al. 2006).

There are many pharmacist-led drug information centers providing services aimed at increasing drug awareness, promoting reasonable prescribing practices, and reducing drug errors.

The pharmacist must practice excellent oral and written communication skills in order to be an effective drug information (DI) provider and be able to:

- Predict and assess patient and healthcare professional DI needs
- Obtain suitable and complete background information

- Analyze and critically assess the literature
- Synthesize, interact with, record, and apply relevant information to the situation in which patients are treated
- Deliver DI to patients, caregivers, and healthcare professionals (Wang et al. 2006).

1.3.2. Self-Care Model

The World Health Organization (WHO) defines *self-care* as "the ability of individuals, families, and communities to promote health, prevent disease, and maintain health and to cope with illness and disability with or without the support of a health-care provider" (WHO 2009).

Pharmacies undoubtedly manage large numbers of patients seeking help and advice for minor illnesses. To provide self-care, the pharmacist must obtain a sufficiently detailed medication history, address the patient's condition properly, carry out proper screening of specific conditions and disorders without interfering with the authority of the prescriber, provide objective medicinal information, use and interpret supplementary sources of information to meet patient needs, help the patient take appropriate and effective over-the-counter medication, or refer the patient for medical advice when necessary (Rutter 2015).

1.3.3. Clinical Pharmacy Model

Clinical pharmacy is a recent discipline of pharmacy practice, where the focus is diverted from a product-based to a patient-oriented practice (Miller 1981). Clinical pharmacy is defined in various ways, as different academic institutions and pharmaceutical societies have sought to describe it from their own perspectives. The American Society of Clinical Pharmacy (ACCP) stated: "Clinical Pharmacy is a health science discipline in which pharmacists provide patient care that optimizes medication therapy and promotes health and disease prevention" (ACCP 2008). The activities of clinical pharmacists differ, as permitted by the authority in each country, but generally range from a prescription review to the prescription of drugs.

Generally, the tasks of clinical pharmacists include: documenting and recording prescription history, reviewing the medication chart of patients, monitoring adverse effects, tracking drug effectiveness and toxicity, assessing, gathering, using, and presenting information related to drugs, and counseling of patients (Anderson 2002). Clinical pharmacy services can be provided to both clinicians and patients and cover all clinical services including, but not limited to, general surgery, ambulatory care, solid organ transplantation, pediatric and adult oncology and hematology, nephrology, pediatrics, infectious disease, internal medicine, adult surgical/medical ICU, neonatology/pediatric ICU, cardiology, parenteral nutrition, pain management, therapeutic drug monitoring, drug information, anticoagulation services, and investigational drug services.

1.3.4. Pharmaceutical Care Model

Pharmaceutical care is a patient-centered, outcome-oriented pharmacy practice that requires pharmacists to work with patients and healthcare providers to promote health, prevent disease, and evaluate, monitor, initiate, and modify drug use to ensure safe and effective drug therapy regimens (Hepler and Strand 1990). The objective of pharmaceutical care is to provide patients with optimal quality services within the sphere of their health care and to assure their well-being and a positive outcome for their treatment while utilizing existing economic resources.

The pharmacist must use the principle of evidence-based pharmacy in each step during the patient care process. Pharmaceutical care steps include:

- *Collection:* The pharmacist must ensure that all available patient information is collected with regard to relevant clinical/ drug history and health status.
- *Assessment:* From the perspective of patient health goals, the pharmacist must assess the collected information and analyze the clinical aspects of patient treatment results to identify significant concerns and assure that optimal care is provided.
- *Planning:* The pharmacist must create care plans on an individual basis that are cost-effective and founded on evidence. Pharmacists must coordinate these activities with other healthcare providers, and with the patients and/or caregivers.

- *Implementation:* The pharmacist must implement the care plan in cooperation with the other healthcare providers, and the patient and/or caregiver.
- *Follow-up:* The pharmacist must follow up and evaluate the efficacy of the care plan and and make appropriate adjustments as needed, with the support of the other healthcare providers, and the patient and/or caregiver (JCPP 2014).
- *Documentation:* The care given to the patients must be documented. Documentation is vital to the continuity of care of a patient and demonstrates both the accountability and the service value of the pharmacist.

1.3.5. Medication Therapy Management (MTM)

In the United States and United Kingdom, when optimizing patient therapy, pharmacists often refer not to the concept of pharmaceutical care, but to the provision of medication management. Pharmaceutical care and medication therapy management are often used interchangeably, but there are some important differences. Medication therapy management was defined by The American Pharmacists Association (APhA) as a "distinct service or group of services that optimize therapeutic outcomes for individual patients" (Bluml 2005). The five core elements of MTM include: a medication therapy review (MTR), personal medication record (PMR), medication-related action plan (MAP), documentation, and follow-up (Bluml 2005).

The key differences are that with pharmaceutical care as the basis of the practice, in-person appointments are of utmost importance, while with MTM, the practice is more task-based, with emphasis on billing per patient intervention. Moreover, MTM can and may be done over the phone. Thus, MTM is offered as a comprehensive model incorporating pharmaceutical care philosophy, methods of counseling patients, and management of disease in a setting where collaboration among patients, pharmacists, and other healthcare providers is encouraged. The MTM services can occur in conjugation with or independent of providing a drug product. The elements of the pharmaceutical care model include a philosophy (Burns 2005), which is its foundation and which forms the basis for the method and the management system of the practice. The MTM, on the other hand, lacks a philosophy and relates to a management operating system having a documenting framework (APhA 2013; McGivney et al. 2007; Whalen 2018.).

1.3.6. Distributive Practice Model

This model is one in which pharmacists mainly distribute medicines and process new orders. The function of a pharmacist is reactive, in that he or she reacts to the doctors' and nurses' requests, with substantial medication adjustments rarely allowed. Pharmacists are not engaged with the healthcare team or in the creation of patient treatment decisions. Subsequently, they are not held responsible for patient health outcomes and impose no influence in guiding the process of drug usage (Holdford and Brown 2010).

1.4. The Nine-Star Pharmacist Concept

- *Caregiver:* The nine star pharmacist concept is a milestone in terms of setting standards for pharmacists to provide patients with very high-quality pharmaceutical care.
- *Decision Maker:* Pharmacists must be focused on specific decisions made or taken to ensure that resources such as personnel, equipment, chemical supplies, medicines, practices and procedures, etc. are used in an appropriate, efficient, secure, and cost-effective manner. Pharmacists also need to play a pivotal role in developing medicine policies at both the local and national levels. The pharmacist must therefore be capable of evaluating and synthesizing information and data and making decisions on the most suitable course of action, i.e., creating hospital formulary following the selection and evaluation of medical agents and their dosage forms which are considered the most useful and pharmaco-economic in patient care (Wright et al. 2019).

- *Communicator:* The pharmacist must create a connection between doctors, patients, and other health care professionals. The development of positive and productive relationships requires both written and verbal communication skills. Included in the care and education of patients are effective techniques which pharmacists can apply to boost patient compliance during drug therapy (Bond 1984). Furthermore, as well as by communicating verbally, improved drug therapy and consequent patient compliance can be achieved via accurately written recommendations to the doctors and patients that address problems with the drug therapy (Doucette et al. 2005).
- *Manager:* Pharmacists must be capable of managing natural and commercial resources, including personnel and physical and financial resources. It is important to take greater responsibility for managing the information on the medication label, maintaining medication health, and preserving professional integrity and practice in patient care activities. The pharmacist must effectively manage departmental policies, procedures, priorities, goals, quality assurance systems, and requirements for environmental health and infection control within his/her institution (Thamby and Parasuraman 2014; Prasad and Tavva 2014). In a community pharmacy, for example, as a manager he/she is responsible for the running of various aspects of the pharmacy such as finances, staff, marketing, sales, and customer services.
- *Lifelong Learner:* In general, a lifelong learner is in "pursuit of awareness in an ongoing, voluntary, and self-motivated basis, for personal or professional purposes" (Ates and Alsal 2012). This therefore promotes not only social inclusion, active citizenship, and personal development, but also self-sustainability, productivity, and employability as well. Lifelong learning concepts must start from the pharmacy school days, and must be promoted throughout the professional life of the pharmacist. Pharmacists regularly update their knowledge and skills to compete with current trends in drug therapy management-related issues (Thamby and Parasuraman

2014; Prasad and Tavva 2014). Guidelines are changeable and knowledge can change as well.

- *Teacher:* One of the duties of a pharmacist is to assist in educating and preparing future generations of pharmacists and the general public. Even community pharmacists play a great role in the pharmacy students' education and training. Community pharmacists can act as preceptors to help students maintain self-confidence and instill responsibility in their profession (Thamby and Parasuraman 2014; Prasad and Tavva 2014).
- *Leader:* Leadership is the practice of inspiring a group of people to take action to achieve a common purpose (Northouse 2007). The skills required for any leadership include effective communication skills, integrative judgment, optimal listening skills, and forward thinking. The pharmacist must play a leadership role in the healthcare system using effective decision-making, communication, and management skills. The power and authority of a leader may be either officially or unofficially acquired. By acquiring experience and skills, young pharmacists become potential informal leaders.
- *Researcher:* Research is important for the pharmacy sector as the results can affect all healthcare sectors. Research should be an integral part of the pharmacist's daily routine. There are many fields in which pharmacists can incorporate research, including pharmaceutical development, rational drug therapy, novel preparation, and preclinical and clinical studies. Pharmacy studies must incorporate community pharmacists along with pharmacist in hospitals, industry, and primary care.

Some foundations have defined research in pharmacy practice. The Canadian Association of Pharmacists has stated: "Research in pharmacy practice is a portion of health services research that focuses on pharmacy practice assessment and evaluation", while the King's Fund 1977 described pharmacy practice research as "research which attempts to inform and understand pharmacy and the way in which it is practiced, in order to support the objectives of pharmacy practice and to ensure that pharmacists' knowledge and

Addressing the Gap between Pharmacy Education and Practice

skills are used to best effect in solving the problems of the health service and meeting the health needs of the population". While the concept of the King's Fund defines large-scale research activity, the Canadian Association of Pharmacists' definition applies to very small-scale projects (CPA n.d.; Toklu 2015).

- *Pharmapreneur:* An entrepreneur is "a person who organizes and operates a business or businesses, taking on greater than normal financial risks in order to do so." The Pharmapreneur is a very new concept which is not adequately represented in the pharmacy sector as most pharmacists prefer to work in already existing institutions such as a community pharmacy or hospital. There are many opportunities in the pharmacy sector that enable the pharmacist to be a great pharmacy entrepreneur. To be a pharmapreneur, a pharmacist must:
    - Possess and apply appropriate knowledge of the pharmaceutical sciences
    - Carry out pharmacist-led patient care
    - Be a lifelong learner, as rules and policies continue to change (Sam and Parasuraman 2015)
    - Create new paradigms for improving outcomes of patient care
    - Produce innovative new pharmaceutical business solutions which enhance patient adherence and strengthen the community pharmacy business.

Does the pharmacist graduated from a School of Pharmacy have those talents and qualifications?

2. PHARMACY EDUCATION

2.1. Different Modules in Pharmacy Education

In most countries, pharmacy education requires four years of courses and one year of pre-registration training. During these courses students learn about the fundamentals of the pharmaceutical sciences. Students can learn from related fields, including medicine, chemistry, genetics, and even ethics. During the final years of study, the approach switches from the theoretical to the practical, which includes conducting an independent research project.

However, many countries have begun to introduce the degree of Doctor of Pharmacy (PharmD), which includes six years of pharmacy education. The PharmD is a professional doctorate degree, also known as a clinical doctorate–a term only used in the health professions. This degree is completely different from the PhD (Doctor of Philosophy) which is used mainly in the academic field (Pierce and Peyton 1999). The new curriculum for the PharmD requires a two-year pre-pharmacy course and four years of practical experience in pharmacy.

In the past, the practice of pharmacy was largely focused on medicine compounding and related services. More recently, in the West, the practice has been moving forward in a more progressive direction, especially in the area of education and qualifications at the university level. In Europe, requirements for professional registration with the relevant pharmacy regulatory board include Master of Pharmacy (MPharm), Bachelor of Science (BSc), or Bachelor of Pharmacy (BPharm) degrees. The regulatory authority for pharmacists, pharmacy technicians, and pharmacy facilities in Britain is the General Pharmaceutical Council (GPhC), which also contributes to pharmacy education by establishing educational standards, authorizing qualifications, and accrediting university pharmacy training programs. The MPharm curriculum incorporates the pharmaceutical sciences into clinical pharmacy practice, which requires a two-year pre-pharmacy course and four years of practical experience in pharmacy (Babar et al. 2019). The BPharm requires four years of education in Australia and five years in Europe. Its equivalent is the MPharm in the United Kingdom. There are still significant gaps in pharmacist education and training within the European Union. In the Netherlands, for example, it takes six years to become a pharmacist, within which no pre-register training is required. Conversely, a practical training period of six months is conducted during the final year of pharmacy school. Two pharmacy credentials are provided by the Scandinavian countries of Norway, Sweden, and Finland. The Pharmacy

Master's degree takes five to six years to complete and requires six months of practical experience in a pharmacy (Mason, 2000). The other credential is the Pharmacy Bachelor's degree, which takes three years to complete.

In Hong Kong, the BPharm is awarded on completion of at least three / four years of full-time study. To be eligible for registration with the Hong Kong Pharmacy and Poisons Board as a practitioner, the applicant must undergo another year of pre-registration training as recommended by the Board.

In the Middle East, the Bachelor's degree in Pharmacy was the first professional degree to be implemented in most of these countries and at least five countries now offer PharmD degree programs. Bachelor's degree programs are usually five years in length across all nations. Pre-pharmacy training (i.e., non-professional years) for Bachelor's degree programs varies in length from 1-2 years (Kheir et al. 2008).

Over the past 200 years, Pharmacy education as well as post-graduate training have changed dramatically in the United States (Hepler, 1987; Higby, 1997; Holland and Nimmo, 1999). The transformation began in the1960s with the introduction of new drug delivery approaches. At the same time, recording of drug histories, patient consultations, and other such clinical pharmacy services were initiated, particularly in pharmacies of larger teaching hospitals. The post-graduate programs established for BSc and doctoral degrees in Pharmacy in the 1970s and 80s boosted the movement toward continuing education and training. By the end of the 1990s, almost 80 accredited pharmacy colleges had begun to adopt the PharmD as the degree required for entrance into the profession in the US.

3. BRIDGING THE GAP BETWEEN EDUCATION AND PRACTICE

Though significant changes are taking place in educational methods, these changes are not sufficient to bridge the gap between education and practice. First of all there is a great deal of debate related to the quality of education, opportunities, and environments for clinical learning experiences, job opportunities, and professional inequalities (Anderson et al. 2012).

Clinical pharmacy nowadays dominates the world's main practice mode and yet many schools continue to deal superficially with clinical pharmacy. Therefore, the graduate pharmacist has difficulty answering patient questions related to many topics such as nuclear pharmacy, complementary medicine, nutraceuticals, homeopathy, and others (Fathelrahman et al. 2016). It has become apparent that pharmacy education needs to respond to professional and social changes and to renew its mission in terms of students and learning objectives.

3.1. Needs-Based Education

"In theory, there is no difference between theory and practice, but in practice there is" stated Manfred Eigen. This disparity can be overcome by analyzing the practice needs. Needs-based education is a strategy which requires any given system to assess its community's needs and then improve (or adapt) the supporting education system accordingly.

Pharmacists have been more engaged in the compounding and manufacturing of medicines in the past century, but over time this position has diminished considerably, and the introduction of the pharmacist into direct patient care has become mandatory. This progress in the position of pharmacists enables them to become part of the broader healthcare team working to provide patients with better healthcare, thus contributing to the achievement of the global Millennium Development Goals. Numerous literature studies support the proposition to involve pharmacists in inter-professional primary health care teams. The pharmacy educational institutions in many countries still have not recognized or continue to ignore the changes in the practice.

Pharmacy institutions should carry out advanced research to determine the needs and promote and support the practice. Country-based research will help confirm whether the education and training system obtained by pharmacy students is good enough to promote positive attitudes and potential integration into primary healthcare. Curricula should better reflect the wide range of career paths potential pharmacists must take in the ever-changing health systems and prepare our students for the many opportunities in pharmacy (DiPiro 2011).

There is a growing challenge to switch from curricula focused on knowledge and skills to curricula that will develop pharmacists as individuals who will, "think, act, and do things in a way that demonstrates they are genuinely patient-centered pharmacists" (Noble et al. 2011).

To overcome the need in many countries, establishing clinical pharmacy specializations is also a current topic of research.

3.2. Changes Needed in the Education Process

3.2.1. Creating Clear and Compelling Outcomes Based on Previous Analyses

Depending on the analytical results, certain outcome for education must be introduced. In 2013, The American Center for the Advancement of Pharmacy Education (CAPE) created educational outcomes for directing instructional and curriculum preparation based on a country-based analysis, and faculty and preceptors discussed the provision of the curriculum accordingly. Four domains were determined by CAPE for the outcomes, which define certain learning objectives that are considered as the gold standard for developing an education syllabus (Piascik 2013):

- Foundational knowledge
- Essentials for practice and care
- Approach to practice
- Personal and professional development

3.2.2. Standardizing Education Based on These Outcomes

Standardization plays a critical role in creating effective national and even international curriculum goals that help prepare pharmacists for the demands in each country and worldwide. Standardization sets clear and measurable goals in the form of instruction and helps measure the outcomes.

3.2.3. Improving Training (Apprenticeship) Programs

The enhancement of the training program should not be limited to increasing the number of training courses, but should extend to the quality of its content. Simulation training can play an important role in upscaling and enhancing pharmacy learning productivity and overcoming the barrier of limited real-field settings. The disparity between community-based and hospital-based training and the courses attributed to graduates must be reduced to provide harmony between pharmacy education and training. The most important skills involve patient care, and these skills come from structured training and experience.

Challenges have been encountered in the past with attempts to develop partnerships between pharmacy schools and university medical centers. Unfortunately, the opportunity to provide an ideal training situation for pharmacy students has been missed due to lack of a mutual understanding. In some cases, students are seen as disrupting elements in the delivery of clinical services because of the time needed to train these students. Clinicians may consider the time spent in student teaching as an obstacle to carrying out their own patient care obligations. Thus, in addition to time spent with patients, the clinicians must be given time to carry out duties in training programs. These training programs have many advantages, including:

- Allowing the students access to students in other areas such as nursing and medicine, and interaction with junior practitioners.
- Acquainting the students with with the processes and procedures of the institution by rotating their duties, and with each rotation, enabling them them to undertake added patient care responsibilities.
- Alleviating time pressure on clinical pharmacists by assigning specific duties such as recording drug histories to students.
- Providing a pool of applicants for residency programs in Pharmacy and entry-level pharmacist positions who are better prepared to play

a direct role in patient care. This can be achieved by incorporating the students into the pharmacy practice model and developing their range of experiences. Thus, the initial investment in providing this preparation can be compensated. However, for this model to be effective, the health system and the pharmacy schools must maintain a close and on-going collaboration.

3.2.4. Introducing Inter-Professional Education (IPE) into the Curriculum

The definition of interdisciplinary/interprofessional education is "the provision of healthcare by providers from various professions in a coordinated way that meets patient needs." Providers share mutual goals, resources and patient care obligations. In clinical practice, it is defined by the term *interprofessional,* whereas the word *interdisciplinary* is often used to describe the educational process (ACCP 2009).

The ignoring of the role of the pharmacist in direct patient care by other health care providers is one of the major obstacles to the success of the pharmacist in providing primary healthcare. Inter-professional education (IPE) prepares students for collaborative thinking and practice. Building this collaborative project through education has a major impact on bridging the gaps between different providers of primary health care (El-Awaisi et al. 2019; Patel et al. 2016).

Collaborative learning is an important tool for promoting health professional education, and has been promoted for many years by many academic institutions, mostly through interprofessional training. Interprofessional education occurs when students from two or more professions learn from each other to work together efficiently and improve health outcomes (WHO, 2015). Many benefits of IPE can be listed:

- Learning with other students will help the pharmacist become a productive member of a healthcare team.
- Differences in educational methods allow a mutually beneficial educational experience to be created.

- Differences in the fields of knowledge and training can bridge the gap between research and practice.
- Ultimately, patients will benefit if healthcare students collaborate to solve patient problems.
- Shared learning between students of different healthcare branches will improve the pharmacists' understanding of clinical problems.
- Studying together with other healthcare students before qualification will improve relations after qualification.
- Communication skills will be more effective if learned with other students in healthcare.
- Studying with students of other healthcare disciplines helps the pharmacist have a positive attitude toward other professionals.
- Studying with students of other healthcare disciplines assists pharmacists in recognizing their own limitations.
- Interprofessional learning plays a role in research production.

Limited financial resources continue to plague healthcare facilities and educational institutions as they seek to fully achieve their goals. As well as the need to care for more patients by working more quickly and more effectively, there is a need to conduct research to improve approaches to patient care.

One technique for overcoming limited resources is to establish alliances with different professionals in the field. The advantages of this approach include a broader perspective when conducting research, the development of new or enhanced clinical knowledge and professional collaborative practices in the clinical and science sectors, and a greater understanding and respect for the professional roles of others (Fauchald and Smith 2005).

"A team of experts does not make an expert team" – and there are a number of obstacles that impede the progress towards IPE including:

- Siloed training and learning
- Lack of common vocabulary across professions
- Disconnecting changes in healthcare provision and education

Addressing the Gap between Pharmacy Education and Practice   19

- Challenges in hiring, training, and supporting creative faculty / preceptors
- Organizational barriers, including finding meeting venues and scheduling of events, timetable differences, and resource deficits
- School or faculty barriers
- Lack of incentive to change
- Lack of knowledge and skills to teach IPE and to practice teamwork
- The time required to implement and change activities (Wilkes 2017).

E-learning may serve as a solution. E-learning aims to overcome some of the logistical challenges of delivering IPE by bringing together students who are located on different campuses for classroom instruction and clinical training. Online learning not only helps to address many of the functional difficulties of IPE, but it also provides a unique forum for developing a digital learning system that can be exported to other institutions.

3.2.5. *Continuing Professional Development (CPD) to Enhance the Workforce*

The healthcare environment is undergoing rapid transformation, and the pharmacist's role is undergoing change. It is now expected that pharmacy graduates will be involved in directly managing patient care via a clinical practice, conducting extensive management of medication, and providing services for preventive care. Continuing education and development at the postgraduate level can prepare pharmacists to prevail over these prospective challenges (Wheeler and Chisholm-Burns 2018).

For decades, the literature has discussed the effect of continuing education on the health professions (Summerlin 2018). Between 1977 and 2014, 39 systematic reviews on the effects of continuing medical education (CME) were published. Such reviews have consistently shown that CME is effective on provider awareness and successful patient outcomes (Cervero and Gaines 2015).

Many nations, including Australia, Canada, New Zealand, and the UK, have adopted the CPD method as a condition for pharmacist re-licensure

(Tran et al. 2014). For example, the Pharmacy Board of Australia requires pharmacists to complete tasks with an aggregate value of 40 or more CPD credits per annum (Pharmacy Board of Australia n.d.).

The structure of the CPD practice for New Zealand pharmacists allows participants to gain "points" from activities in three distinct learning groups: activities with minimal or no attendant interaction, activities with knowledge acquisition checked through evaluation, and programs based on practical changes defined through reflection and supporting evidence of practical outcomes (Pharmaceutical Society of New Zealand n.d.).

In the United Kingdom, the General Pharmaceutical Council operates an online system for the exchange of CPD records online with managers or other colleagues who help or track CPD activities (General Pharmaceutical Council n.d.).

Effective CPD faces many obstacles. There is a need to develop CPD models that remove barriers, optimize efficiencies, and reduce the burden. Using technology to promote learning can mitigate specific obstacles such as travel funding and time lost. Learner groups with shared interests can be developed to foster creativity and support sustainability. Simulation is likely to play a greater role in CPD, particularly if a large number of practitioners need to reorganize their skills set to assume direct roles in patient care (Sachdeva 2016). The main elements of CPD include:

- Reflecting: Self-assessment of the needs or priorities of staff or institution,
- Planning: Identifying goals, creating opportunities for formal and informal learning, identifying measures of success, and articulating strategy with colleagues,
- Learning: Implementing of designed programs,
- Evaluating: Assessing the quality of learning and its effects on success and related outcomes (Wheeler and Chisholm-Burns 2018).

3.2.6. Incorporating New Education Methodologies, Technologies, and Simulation in Pharmacy Education

The Pharmacy School student nowadays is typically from Generation Z. This generation relies greatly on technology and tends to embrace hands-on social learning environments where they can be involved directly in the learning process. They expect services on demand that can be accessed at any time, with few obstructions. Moreover, they seem to be more career-oriented at their colleges (Cilliers 2017). The method of education must be adapted to suit the demands of this generation. Hence, different types of education methodology must be incorporated into the pharmacy syllabus. Some of these approaches include:

- *Interactive lectures:* The instructor interrupts the lecture at least once per class to have students participate in an activity that allows them to work directly with the material. This leads to improved teacher/student and student/student interactions. Active participation can be encouraged and the value of lecture sessions enhanced by think-pair-sharing, practical demonstrations, role-playing, and other similar techniques. Active learning strategies include team-based and problem-based learning (Gleason et al. 2011).
- *Team-based learning:* This is a structured form of small-group learning that emphasizes class preparation and application of knowledge in the classroom. Students are strategically organized into diverse teams of 5–7 students working together throughout the course. Students prepare by reading prior to class before each unit or module of the course (Farland et al. 2013).
- *Problem-based learning (PBL):* Students are engaged in a problem and a series of progressive misunderstandings triggers the identification of gaps in their knowledge which require more self-directed learning. Students have the chance to create educational goals, and PBL helps students to improve problem-solving skills, self-directed learning, and collaboration and to enhance their intrinsic motivation (Galvao et al. 2014).

- *Case-based learning (CBL):* The CBL approach is more structured than PBL, and is generally used in pharmacotherapy classes. In CBL, the exact problem of the case is provided in detail, while in problem-based learning the students must determine the problem by themselves (Thistlethwaite et al. 2012).
- *Simulation-based training (SBT):* For several decades, state-of-the-art simulation-based training has been extensively used in healthcare. The variety of simulation tools currently available to support skill development includes patient and computer-based simulations and virtual reality simulations. This type of training provides a safe environment in which pharmacists can improve their professional skills and develop other technical and non-technical abilities, such as communication skills, collaboration techniques, and proficiency in decision-making and the prioritization of tasks. This approach helps in the preparation of individual or multiprofessional teams and provides the capability for increased team performance and patient safety.

Didactic learning is not enough to deal with emergencies or unusual health conditions (Sarfati et al. 2018). By comparison, SBT can deliver a rich educational forum focused on learners and provide meaningful experiences to ready participants for managing any emergency situation.

Types of Simulation

Health education can benefit from the extensive range of simulation tools available to support learning, critical thinking and clinical skills. These include devices used in acquiring drug administration and emergency management skills. Examples of those used in SBT are patient simulations, virtual reality (VR) patients, and computer-based learning simulations (Cavaco and Madeira 2012; Aebersold 2016). In the case of standardized patients, scenarios or clinical conditions are modeled by lay persons, actors, faculty members, or student peers. Students follow a structured sequence of scenarios and communicate through the computers or VR headsets in computer-based education systems and VR simulators. The decision-making skills of pharmacy students are improved via self-directed learning in one oncology pharmaco-therapeutics program using computer-based simulation (Bernaitis et al. 2018). In addition, accuracy in the documentation of medical notes is evaluated and supported by the use of simulated electronic patient records. A full range of SBT types is available, including those using patient simulations where low- to high-fidelity scenarios can be performed *in situ* or in a clinical setting.

> ***High-fidelity SBT:*** The effectiveness of the use of high-fidelity simulation in pharmacy schools has been highly promising in the USA, while data in other countries are limited (Stockert et al. 2008; Regan et al. 2014). Through the evolving computer software and technology, some of the more sophisticated high-fidelity mannequins currently available for healthcare training can speak, breathe, and generate realistic heart and lung sounds, and many also include more complex configurations for the enhancement of the learner experience by mimicking physiological reactions to procedures and treatment, including physiological responses to drug administration. Examples include the programmable SimMan ® 3 G (Laerdal Medical; see Figure 2), Human Patient Simulator (METI) and Emergency Care Simulator (METI).
>
> ***Simulation Software***: This is used efficiently by some schools of pharmacy, and the positive impact of this software on the education outcomes has been reported by many pharmacy schools.
>
> ***Mydispense***: Monash University has developed this software that enables students to build competencies and trust during pharmaceutical dispensing. Mydispense is a web application that facilitates a complete dispensing experience, from initial patient and prescriber contact to professional advice when dispensing medications to patients. This software incorporates a dispensing framework with many characteristics of commercial dispensing systems to provide students with authentic experience of current dispensing practices. The students receive rich, detailed feedback on

their dispensing performance at the end of each exercise (McDowell et al. 2016).

Pharmatopia Program: Monash University also developed this interactive simulation program which is an online learning platform where students experience the process of making tablets (Duncan and Larson 2012).

Pharmville: This is a teaching tool that presents patients with real problems to provide meaning and integration throughout the undergraduate program. Each character in Pharmville has a distinct cultural and social context, lifestyle, and medical history. Faculty and staff across all disciplines can use Pharmville as a framework to engage students in principles of science and professional practice, relating theory directly to real circumstances, including individuals, families and communities (Marriott et al. 2012). The content platform includes video vignettes, character portraits, photos of the drug system, recorded health records, and medical and social backgrounds. This promotes and supports the application of the principles of the coursework to individuals, and provides more meaning to teaching.

Challenges and Limitations of SBT

- SBT is an add-on tool and not a replacement for clinical experience, and its mimicking of human systems is incomplete.
- SBT comes at high cost. Capacity to house a simulation suite is required along with qualified personnel. The position and role of SBT in any pharmacy curriculum needs to be defined and coordinated with relevant skills.
- The effect on both educational and clinical results needs more study and validation (Lloyd et al. 2018).

Technological Approaches: The students must engage in education that supports their proper use of certain technology. Generally, technology is incorporated in pharmacy through the infrastructure (e.g., mobile computing, telemedicine, remote systems, robotic devices), business operations and rules (e.g., medication purchasing and financial processes, regulatory requirements), the medication order entry process (e.g., computerized provider order entry [CPOE]), ePrescribing, medication dispensing and distribution (e.g., robotics), medication administration (e.g., intravenous smart pumps, bar code administration, radio frequency identification), and information storage, retrieval, evaluation, and dissemination.

3.2.7. *Implementing Curricular Integration in Pharmacy Education*

Curricular integration has been defined as the "intentional uniting or meshing of discrete elements or features (of a planned educational experience" (Case 1991). An integrated curriculum is known to have horizontal and vertical dimensions. Horizontal integration in pharmacy programs usually refers to integration across basic science disciplines such as medical chemistry, pharmaceutics and pharmacology, while vertical integration typically refers to basic and clinical science integration (Brueckner and Gould 2006). A comprehensive approach to developing an integrated pharmacy program needs to address both horizontal and vertical dimensions as well as systemic and pedagogical approaches to promote integrative learning.

Vertical integration is the connection across time and between theory and practice. Vertical integration has two elements: (1) the progression of the curriculum over time, where content unfolds in a logical order and prior learning is taken into account and used to benefit and (2) the connection to real-world contexts where learning is applied.

A more progressive approach is the system of "inverted triangles", with clinical experience offered from the start and slowly becoming more dominant and with the fundamental sciences dominant in the beginning and persisting until the end of the program (Dooley-Hash 2010). The purpose of this curriculum framework is to improve the convergence of theory and practice by using early clinical experience and fostering a grounding in the basic sciences of clinical practice.

As with any significant curricular reform, there are many obstacles to be faced while developing an integrated curriculum. For example, considerable time and effort is required to develop a cohesive study program to promote the development of higher-order student knowledge, skills, and abilities (Pearson and Hubball 2012).

3.2.8. Initiating Effective Collaboration
"One Hand Can't Clap Alone"

Pharmacy education is a focus field for the International Pharmaceutical Federation (FIP), the worldwide multinational federation of pharmacists and pharmaceutical scientists heading the Multinational Pharmacy Education Taskforce. Organizations such as WHO and the United Nations Educational, Scientific, and Cultural Organization (UNESCO) have played a great role in defining the standards for pharmacy education. Working together with such organizations will provide for the globalization of this field.

Great efforts must be made to assert strategic leadership and optimize the effect of collective action between these organizations and academic institutions at global, regional, and national levels. Globalization brings with it the internationalization of education as universities broaden their borders beyond traditional countries or regional boundaries and populations strive to move more freely between countries (Lee 2011).

REFERENCES

ACCP (The American Society of Clinical Pharmacy). 2008. "The Definition of Clinical Pharmacy." *Pharmacotherapy* 28(6): 816–817. https://doi.org/10.1592/phco.28.6.816.

ACCP (The American Society of Clinical Pharmacy). 2009. "ACCP White Paper, Interprofessional Education: Principles and Application. A Framework for Clinical Pharmacy" *Pharmacotherapy* 29:148e-164e.

Aebersold, Michelle. 2016. "The History of Simulation and Its Impact on the Future." *AACN Advanced Critical Care* 27(1): 56–61. https://doi.org/10.4037/aacnacc2016436.

Anderson, Claire, Bates, Ian, Brock, Tina, Brown, Andrew N., Bruno, Andreia, Futter, Billy, Rennie, Timothy and Rouse, Michael J. 2012. "Needs-Based Education in the Context of Globalization." *American Journal of Pharmaceutical Education* 76(4): 56. https://doi.org/10.5688/ajpe76456.

Anderson, Stuart. 2002. "The State of the World's Pharmacy: A Portrait of the Pharmacy Profession." *Journal of Interprofessional Care* 16(4): 391–404. https://doi.org/10.1080/1356182021000008337.

APhA (The American Pharmacists Association). 2013. "Medication Therapy Management (MTM)." *APhA Foundation* https://www.aphafoundation.org/medication-therapy-management.

Ates, Haydar, and Alsal, Kadir. 2012. "The Importance of Lifelong Learning Has Been Increasing." *Procedia - Social and Behavioral Sciences* 46: 4092–4096. https://doi.org/10.1016/j.sbspro.2012.06.205.

Babar, Zaheer-ud-din, Awaisu, Ahmed, and Chen, Timothy. 2019. *Encyclopedia of Pharmacy Practice and Clinical Pharmacy*. Amsterdam: Elsevier.

Bernaitis, Nijole, Baumann-Birkbeck, Lyndsee, Alcorn, Sean, Powell, Michael, Arora, Devinder, and Anoopkumar-Dukie, Shailendra. 2018. "Simulated Patient Cases Using DecisionSim™ Improves Student Performance and Satisfaction in Pharmacotherapeutics Education." *Currents in Pharmacy Teaching and Learning* 10(6): 730–735. https://doi.org/10.1016/j.cptl.2018.03.020.

Bluml, Benjamin M. 2005. "Definition of Medication Therapy Management: Development of Professionwide Consensus." *Journal of the American Pharmacists Association* 45(5): 566–572. https://doi.org/10.1331/1544345055001274.

Bond, C. A. 1984. "Sustained Improvement in Drug Documentation, Compliance, and Disease Control. A Four-Year Analysis of an Ambulatory Care Model." *Archives of Internal Medicine* 144(6): 1159–1162. https://doi.org/10.1001/archinte.144.6.1159.

Borchardt, John K. 2002. "The Beginnings of Drug Therapy: Ancient Mesopotamian Medicine." *Drug News & Perspectives* 15(3): 187-192.

Brueckner, Jennifer K., and Gould, Douglas J. 2006. "Health science faculty members' perceptions of curricular integration: Insights and obstacles." *Journal of the International Association of Medical Science Educators* 16(1): 31-34.

Burns, Anne. 2005. "Medication Therapy Management in Community Pharmacy Practice: Core Elements of an MTM Service (Version 1.0)." *Journal of the American Pharmacists Association* 45(5): 573–579. https://doi.org/10.1331/1544345055001256.

Case, R. 1991. "The anatomy of curricular integration." Canadian Journal of Education 16(2):215-224.

Cavaco, Afonso Miguel, and Madeira, Filipe. 2012. "European Pharmacy Students Experience with Virtual Patient Technology." *American Journal of Pharmaceutical Education* 76(6): 106. https://doi.org/10.5688/ajpe766106.

Cervero, Ronald M., and Gaines, Julie K. 2015. "The Impact of CME on Physician Performance and Patient Health Outcomes: An Updated Synthesis of Systematic Reviews." *Journal of Continuing Education in the Health Professions* 35(2): 131–138. https://doi.org/10.1002/chp.21290.

Cilliers, Elizelle Juaneé. 2017. "The challenge of teaching generation Z." *PEOPLE: International Journal of Social Sciences* 3(1): 188-198.

CPA (Canadian Pharmacists Association). n.d. Accessed February 26, 2020. http://www.pharmacists.ca/education-practice-resources/pharmacy-practice-research/.

Dipiro, Joseph T. 2011. "Preparing Our Students for the Many Opportunities in Pharmacy." *American Journal of Pharmaceutical Education* 75(9): 170. https://doi.org/10.5688/ajpe759170.

Dooley-Hash, Suzanne. 2010. "Educating Physicians: A Call for Reform of Medical School and Residency." *JAMA* 304(11): 1240. https://doi.org/10.1001/jama.2010.1351.

Doucette, William R., Mcdonough, Randal P., Klepser, Donald, and McCarthy, Renee. 2005. "Comprehensive Medication Therapy Management: Identifying and Resolving Drug-Related Issues in a

Community Pharmacy." *Clinical Therapeutics* 27(7): 1104–1111. https://doi.org/10.1016/s0149-2918(05)00146-3.

Duncan, Gregory, Larson, Ian. 2012. "Professional Education Using E-Simulations." *Advances in Mobile and Distance Learning* https://doi.org/10.4018/978-1-61350-189-4.

El-Awaisi, Alla, Joseph, Sundari, El Hajj, Maguy Saffouh, and Diack, Lesley. 2019. "Pharmacy Academics' Perspectives toward Interprofessional Education Prior to Its Implementation in Qatar: A Qualitative Study." *BMC Medical Education* 19(1) https://doi.org/10.1186/s12909-019-1689-5.

Farland, Michelle Z., Sicat, Brigitte L., Franks, Andrea S., Pater, Karen S., Medina, Melissa S., and Persky, Adam M. 2013. "Best Practices for Implementing Team-Based Learning in Pharmacy Education." *American Journal of Pharmaceutical Education* 77(8): 177. https://doi.org/10.5688/ajpe778177.

Fathelrahman, Ahmed Ibrahim, Ibrahim, Mohamed I.M., and Wertheimer, Albert I. 2016. *Pharmacy Practice in Developing Countries: Achievements and Challenges*. Amsterdam: Elsevier/AP.

Fauchald, Sally K., and Smith, Dave. 2005. "Transdisciplinary research partnerships: Making research happen!" *Nursing Economics* 23(3): 131.

Galvao, Tais F., Silva, Marcus T., Neiva, Celiane S., Ribeiro, Laura M., and Pereira, Mauricio G. 2014. "Problem-Based Learning in Pharmaceutical Education: A Systematic Review and Meta-Analysis." *The Scientific World Journal* 2014 (3): 578382. https://doi.org/10.1155/2014/578382.

Gleason, Brenda L., Peeters, Michael J., Resman-Targoff, Beth H., Karr, Samantha, Mcbane, Sarah, Kelley, Kristi, Thomas, Tyan, and Denetclaw, Tina H.2011. "An Active-Learning Strategies Primer for Achieving Ability-Based Educational Outcomes." *American Journal of Pharmaceutical Education* 75(9): 186. https://doi.org/10.5688/ajpe759186.

Hepler, Charles D. 1987. "The third wave in pharmaceutical education: The clinical movement." *Journal of Pharmaceutical Education* 51(4): 369-385.

Hepler, Charles D., and Strand, Linda M. 1990. "Opportunities and Responsibilities in Pharmaceutical Care." *American Journal of Health-System Pharmacy* 47(3): 533–543. https://doi.org/10.1093/ajhp/47.3.533.

Higby, Gregory J. 1997. *The Inside Story of Medicines: A Symposium.* Madison, WI: American Institute of the History of Pharmacy.

Holdford, David A., and Brown, Thomas R., eds. 2010. *Introduction to Hospital and Health-System Pharmacy Practice.* ASHP.

Holland, Ross W., and Nimmo, Christine M. 1999. "Transitions in Pharmacy Practice, Part 3: Effecting Change—the Three-Ring Circus." *American Journal of Health-System Pharmacy* 56(21): 2235–2241. https://doi.org/10.1093/ajhp/56.21.2235.

JCPP (Joint Commission of Pharmacy Practitioners). 2014. https://www.pharmacist.com/sites/default/files/files/PatientCareProcess.pdf.

Kheir, Nadir, Zaidan, Manal, Younes, Husam, El Hajj, Maguy, Wilbur, Kerry, and Jewesson, Peter J. 2008. "Pharmacy Education and Practice in 13 Middle Eastern Countries." *American Journal of Pharmaceutical Education* 72(6): 133. https://doi.org/10.5688/aj7206133.

Kremers, Edward, Urdang, George, and Sonnedecker, Glenn. 1986. *Kremers and Urdang's History of Pharmacy.* Madison, WI: American Institute of the History of Pharmacy.

Lee, Wing On. 2011. "Learning for the Future: the Emergence of Lifelong Learning and the Internationalisation of Education as the Fourth Way?" *Educational Research for Policy and Practice* 11(1): 53–64. https://doi.org/10.1007/s10671-011-9122-9.

Lloyd, Michael, Watmough, Simon, and Bennett, Nicholas. 2018. "Simulation-based training: Applications in clinical pharmacy." *Clinical Pharmacist* 10(9): 3-10. https://doi.org/10.1211/cp.2018.20205302.

Marriott, Jennifer, Styles, Kim, and McDowell, Jenny. 2012. "The Pharmville Community: A Curriculum Resource Platform Integrating Context and Theory." *American Journal of Pharmaceutical Education* 76(9): 178. https://doi.org/10.5688/ajpe769178.

Mason, Mark. 2000. "Teachers as Critical Mediators of Knowledge." *Journal of the Philosophy of Education* 34(2): 343–342. https://doi.org/10.1111/1467-9752.00177.

McDowell, Jenny, Styles, Kim, Sewell, Keith, Trinder, Peta, Marriott, Jennifer, Maher, Sheryl, and Naidu, Som. 2016. "A Simulated Learning Environment for Teaching Medicine Dispensing Skills." *American Journal of Pharmaceutical Education* 80(1): 11. https://doi.org/10.5688/ajpe80111.

McGivney, Melissa Somma, Meyer, Susan M., Duncan–Hewitt, Wendy, Hall, Deanne L., Goode, Jean-Venable R. 2007. "Counseling, Disease Management, and Pharmaceutical Care." *Journal of the American Pharmacists Association* 47(5): 620–628. https://doi.org/10.1331/japha.2007.06129.

Miller, R.R. 1981. "History of Clinical Pharmacy and Clinical Pharmacology." *Clinical Pharmacology* 21: 195-197.

Noble, Christy, Shaw, P. Nicholas, Nissen, Lisa, Coombes, Ian, and Obrien, Mia. 2011. "Curriculum for Uncertainty: Certainty May Not Be the Answer." *American Journal of Pharmaceutical Education* 75(1): 13a. https://doi.org/10.5688/ajpe75113a.

Northouse, G. 2007. *Leadership Theory and Practice*, 3rd ed. Thousand Oaks, CA: Sage Publications.

Patel, Nilesh, Begum, Shahmina, and Kayyali, Reem. 2016. "Interprofessional Education (IPE) and Pharmacy in the UK. A Study on IPE Activities across Different Schools of Pharmacy." *Pharmacy* 4(4): 28. https://doi.org/10.3390/pharmacy4040028.

Pearson, Marion L., and Hubball, Harry T. 2012. "Curricular Integration in Pharmacy Education." *American Journal of Pharmaceutical Education* 76(10): 204. https://doi.org/10.5688/ajpe7610204.

Pharmaceutical Society of New Zealand. *Recertification Framework* (n.d.).

Pharmacy Board of Australia n.d.

Piascik, Peggy. "CAPE Outcomes 2013: Building on Two Decades of Advances to Guide the Future of Pharmacy Education." *American Journal of Pharmaceutical Education* 77, no. 8 (2013): 160. https://doi.org/10.5688/ajpe778160.

Pierce, D., and Peyton, C. 1999. "A Historical Cross-Disciplinary Perspective on the Professional Doctorate in Occupational Therapy." *American Journal of Occupational Therapy* 53(1): 64–71. https://doi.org/10.5014/ajot.53.1.64.

Prasad, Mohanta Guru, and Tavva, Praveen. 2014. "8-Star Pharmacist." *Handbook of Medicine for Pharmacists.* New Delhi, India: Jaypee Brothers Medical Publishers. https://doi.org/10.5005/jp/books/12322_9.

Regan, Kirsty, Harney, Lisa, Goodhand, Kate, Strath, Alison, and Vosper, Helen. 2014. "Pharmacy Simulation: A Scottish, Student-Led Perspective with Lessons for the UK and Beyond." *Pharmacy* 2(1): 50–64. https://doi.org/10.3390/pharmacy2010050.

Rutter, Paul. 2015. "Role of Community Pharmacists in Patients' Self-Care and Self-Medication." *Integrated Pharmacy Research and Practice* 4:57-65. https://doi.org/10.2147/iprp.s70403.

Sachdeva, Ajit K. 2016. "Continuing Professional Development in the Twenty-First Century." *Journal of Continuing Education in the Health Professions* 36: S8-S13. https://doi.org/10.1097/ceh.0000000000000107.

Sam, Aaseer Thamby, and Parasuraman, Subramani. 2015. "The Nine-Star Pharmacist: An Overview." *Journal of Young Pharmacists* 7(4): 281–284. https://doi.org/10.5530/jyp.2015.4.1. http://www.jyoungpharm.org/sites/default/files/10.5530jyp.2015.4.1.pdf.

Sarfati, Laura, Ranchon, Florence, Vantard, Nicolas, Schwiertz, Vérane, Larbre, Virginie, Parat, Stéphanie, Faudel, Amélie, and Rioufol, Catherine. 2018. "Human-Simulation-Based Learning to Prevent Medication Error: A Systematic Review." *Journal of Evaluation in Clinical Practice* 25(1): 11–20. https://doi.org/10.1111/jep.12883.

Stockert, Brad, Brady, Debra, and Kelly, Katherine. 2008. "The Use of Human Patient Simulators to Train Physical Therapy Students for Work in Critical Care Settings." *Cardiopulmonary Physical Therapy Journal* 19(4): 133–134. https://doi.org/10.1097/01823246-200819040-00031.

Summerlin, Charles. 2019. "Preparing the Future Generation of Pharmacists through Postgraduate Training: Lessons Learned and Advice for Current

Student Pharmacists." *Journal of the American Pharmacists Association* 59(1): 7–8. https://doi.org/10.1016/j.japh.2018.11.010.

Taylor, David. 2015. "The Pharmaceutical Industry and the Future of Drug Development." *Issues in Environmental Science and Technology Pharmaceuticals in the Environment*, 1–33. https://doi.org/10.1039/9781782622345-00001.

Thamby, Sam Aaseer, and Parasuraman, Subramani. 2014. "Seven-Star Pharmacist Concept by World Health Organization." *Journal of Young Pharmacists* 6(2): 1–3. https://doi.org/10.5530/jyp.2014.2.1.

Thistlethwaite, Jill Elizabeth, Davies, David, Ekeocha, Samilia, Kidd, Jane M., MacDougall, Colin, Matthews, Paul, Purkis, Judith, and Clay, Diane. 2012. "The Effectiveness of Case-Based Learning in Health Professional Education. A BEME Systematic Review: BEME Guide No. 23." *Medical Teacher* 34(6): e421-e444 https://doi.org/10.3109/0142159x.2012.680939.

Titsingh, Isaac. 1834. *Annales des Empereurs du Japon* [*Annals of the Emperors of Japan*], p. 434.

Toklu, Hale Zerrin, and Hussain, Azhar. 2013. "The Changing Face of Pharmacy Practice and the Need for a New Model of Pharmacy Education." *Journal of Young Pharmacists* 5(2): 38–40. https://doi.org/10.1016/j.jyp.2012.09.001.

Toklu, Hale. 2015. "Promoting Evidence-Based Practice in Pharmacies." *Integrated Pharmacy Research and Practice* 4:127-131. https://doi.org/10.2147/iprp.s70406.

Tran, Deanna, Tofade, Toyin, Thakkar, Namrata, and Rouse, Michael. 2014. "US and International Health Professions' Requirements for Continuing Professional Development." *American Journal of Pharmaceutical Education* 78(6): 129. https://doi.org/10.5688/ajpe786129.

Wang, Fei, Troutman, William G., Seo, Teresa, Peak, Amy, and Rosenberg, Jack M. 2006. "Drug Information Education in Doctor of Pharmacy Programs." *American Journal of Pharmaceutical Education* 70(3): 51. https://doi.org/10.5688/aj700351.

Whalen, Karen. *"Overview of Medication Therapy Management Data Sets." Medication Therapy Management: A Comprehensive Approach.* New York: McGraw-Hill Medical, 2018.

Wheeler, James S., and Chisholm-Burn, Marie. 2018. "The Benefit of Continuing Professional Development for Continuing Pharmacy Education." *American Journal of Pharmaceutical Education* 82(3): 6461. https://doi.org/10.5688/ajpe6461.

WHO (World Health Organization) Regional Office for South-East Asia. 2009. *"Self-care in the Context of Primary Health Care: Report of the Regional Consultation Bangkok, Thailand"*, 7–9 January 2009. New Delhi: WHO Regional Office for South-East Asia. Available at: apps.searo.who.int/PDS_DOCS/B4301.pdf. (Accessed February 26, 2020)

WHO (World Health Organization). 2015. *"Framework for Action on Interprofessional Education and Collaborative Practice."* https://www.who.int/hrh/resources/framework_action/en/.

Wiedenmayer, K., Summers, R., Mackie, C., Gous, A., Everard, M., and Tromp, D. 2006. *Developing Pharmacy Practice: A Focus on Patient Care Handbook.* Geneva/The Hague, The Netherlands: World Health Organization, Department of Medicine Policies and Standards/ Switzerland and International Pharmaceutical Federation.

Wilkes, Michael, and Robin Kennedy. "Interprofessional Health Sciences Education: It's Time to Overcome Barriers and Excuses." *Journal of General Internal Medicine* 32, no. 8 (November 2017): 858–59. https://doi.org/10.1007/s11606-017-4069-z.

Wright, Daniel F.B., Anakin, Megan G., and Duffull, Stephen B. 2019. "Clinical Decision-Making: An Essential Skill for 21st Century Pharmacy Practice." *Research in Social and Administrative Pharmacy* 15(5): 600–606. https://doi.org/10.1016/j.sapharm.2018.08.001.

BIOGRAPHICAL SKETCH

Nilay Aksoy

Affiliation: Altinbas University School of Pharmacy/Clinical Pharmacy Department

Education:
1997-2002	Alazhar University/ Palestine Bachelor of Pharmacy
2006-2008	Alexandria University/Egypt Master Degree in Clinical Pharmacy
2012-2016	Marmara University/Turkey PhD in Clinical Pharmacy

Business Address: Zuhuratbaba, İncirli Cd. No:11-A, 34147 Bakırköy/İstanbul

Research and Professional Experience:
1. "Investigation of pharmacological potential of the gel prepared by Eugenia Jamboolana. in the Experimental Rats Mucositis Model" (BAP project)
2. " Determination of sensitivity of different antibiotics and combinations of antibiotics in staphylococcal biofilm infections in pediatric hematology oncology patients" (BAP project)
3. "The effect of biofilm inhibitors on the minimum inhibitory concentration of antibiotics used in gram negative bacteria in the biofilm structure" (BAP Project)
4. "Determination of potential drug plant interactions in diabetic patients" (Clinical Pharmacy Project in collaboration with 28 pharmacies in Bakırköy and Bahçelievler /Istanbul, on-going)
5. "The effect of cardiovascular drugs on drug complexity and its relationship with drug-induced problems." (Clinical Pharmacy

Project in collaboration with 28 pharmacies in Bakırköy and Bahçelievler /Istanbul, on-going)
6. "Assessment of the level of consciousness for the risk factor of cancer disease in the community." (Clinical Pharmacy Project in collaboration with 28 pharmacies in Bakırköy and Bahçelievler /Istanbul, on-going)
7. "Evaluation of the effects of probiotics on reducing signs and symptoms of ulcerative colitis, Crohn's, and irritable bowel syndrome." (Clinical Pharmacy Project in collaboration with 28 pharmacies in Bakırköy and Bahçelievler /Istanbul, on-going)
8. "Rational use of vitamins in pregnancy." (Clinical Pharmacy Project in collaboration with 28 pharmacies in Bakırköy and Bahçelievler /Istanbul, on-going)
9. "Evaluation of educational needs for diabetic patients." (Clinical Pharmacy Project in collaboration with 28 pharmacies in Bakırköy and Bahçelievler /Istanbul, on-going)

Supervised Master and PhD Theses:
1. "The relationship between monocyte / YDL-C ratio and GWTG-HF risk score in patients with heart failure." PhD thesis, Medipol University Student Büşra Nur Çattık.
2. "Reduction of Colistin-Induced Nephrotoxicity by N-Acetylcysteine in the Intensive Care Unit." PhD thesis. Medipol University Student Gamze Odabaşı.
3. "The role of clinical pharmacist in Community Pharmacy in providing pharmaceutical care for patients with vitamin D deficiency and determining the risk factors." Master Degree thesis. Medipol University Student Cansu Gürol.
4. "Evaluation of drug-related problems among proton pump inhibitors users; Community setting." Master Degree thesis. Clinical Pharmacy, Medipol University Student Saide Ayanoğlu.

Professional Appointments:

2014 – present	Istanbul, Altınbaş University School of Pharmacy, Prof. Mehmet Tanol, mehmet.tanol@altinbas.edu.tr; Head of Clinical Pharmacy Department
2008 – 2010	Palestine, Ministry of Health, Naser Hospital, Clinical Pharmacist
2004 – 2006	Palestine, Ministry Of Health, Naser Hospital, Pharmacist

Publications from the last 3 years:
1. İzzettin, F. V., Çelik, S., Acar, R. D., Tezcan, S., Aksoy, N., Bektay, M. Y., & Sancar, M. (2019). The role of the clinical pharmacist in patient education and monitoring of patients under warfarin treatment. *Marmara Pharmaceutical Journal*, 23(6).
2. Abunahlah, N., Elawaisi, A., Velibeyoglu, F. M., & Sancar, M. (2018). Drug related problems identified by clinical pharmacist at an Internal Medicine ward in Turkey. *International Journal of Clinical Pharmacy*, 40(2), 360-367.
3. Abunahlah, N., Abimbola, A., & Okuturlar, Y. (2017). Use of Heparin and the Related Incidence of Heparin-Induced Thrombocytopenia in an Education and Research Hospital in Turkey. *Journal of Clinical and Experimental Investigations*, 8(3), 71.
4. Abunahlah, N., Sancar, M., Dane, F., & Özyavuz, M. K. (2016). Impact of adherence to antiemetic guidelines on the incidence of chemotherapy-induced nausea and vomiting and quality of life. *J Clin Pharm*, DOI:10.1007/s11096-016-0393-3.

In: Pharmacists
Editor: Line L. Villadsen

ISBN: 978-1-53618-018-3
© 2020 Nova Science Publishers, Inc.

Chapter 2

CURRENT CHALLENGES AND PERSPECTIVES OF PHARMACIST IN ONCOLOGY SETTINGS

Songül Tezcan[*]
Department of Clinical Pharmacy, Marmara University,
Istanbul, Turkey

ABSTRACT

Multidisciplinary approach is one of the corner stones of the successful cancer therapy. Pharmacist as a health advisor in multidisciplinary team has a vital role in oncology setting. The oncology pharmacists (OPs) are the specialist pharmacists on oncology and involved in the planning and administration of chemotherapy, which is the most common cancer treatment.

OPs in the multidisciplinary team contribute to the rational use of chemotherapy and supportive drugs by providing individual pharmaceutical care plans for patients. Pharmaceutical care is a new discipline, which was first defined, by Charles D. Hepler and Linda M. Strand in 1990. The definition of pharmaceutical care has been improved with some changes over time. According to these definitions; the

---

[*] Corresponding Author's Email: songulbutur@hotmail.com.

pharmacist's responsibilities include preventing, identifying and solving the drug related problems (DRPs), providing patient-oriented service, making a care plan, following up patients. Recent studies have shown that pharmaceutical care programs have positive contributions to the treatment of oncology patients.

The increasing incidence of cancer cases and the development of new drugs lead to application of personalized therapies. Many studies have shown that OPs contribute to optimize the medication use and to provide rationale therapy. However, during pharmaceutical care process, OPs sometimes face to challenges with doctors, patients, nurses and other health professionals. This chapter will focus on pharmacist role in oncology and current challenges and perspectives of pharmacist in oncology settings.

Keywords: oncology pharmacists, patient-oriented service, pharmaceutical care, challenges

1. INTRODUCTION

Multidisciplinary approach is an essential method for the management of many chronic diseases, due to the complexity of treatments and difficulties in patient monitoring. Cancer is a chronic disease, which consists of more than 100 different diseases. The disease is characterized by uncontrolled growing of abnormal cells in organs or tissues, local invasion and distant metastasis. Mortality of cancer is increasing in worldwide. It is the second most common cause of deaths after cardiovascular diseases in the United States of America (USA) (American Cancer Society 2019). Over 600,000 cancer-related deaths were reported in the USA, in 2019 (Siegel et al. 2019). In additionally, the prevalence and the incidence of cancer is increasing globally. It has been reported that in 2019, approximately 1,8 million new cancer cases occur in the United States (Siegel et al. 2019).

Along with the increasing prevalence of cancer, the development of new chemotherapeutic agents also continues. Use of chemotherapeutic agents, which started with the use of nitrosoureas in cancer treatment in the early 1940s, has shown a great improvement in recent years with the use of immunological therapies for cancer treatment.

Nowadays, surgery, radiotherapy, systemic chemotherapy, targeted agents and immunological treatments are used alone and/or as combination regimens, in the treatment of cancer (Shord 2014). While advances in treatment continue to promise hope, early diagnosis and prevention of cancer remains to be another strategic point.

In addition to the developments in the field of diagnosis and treatment of cancer, changes in the health system also positively affect the treatment process of cancer. It is an indisputable fact that "multidisciplinary teamwork in cancer therapy" is an essential approach. Pharmacists, involved in the multidisciplinary team, are the closest accessible health consultants and have an essential role in pharmaceutical services by changing drug-oriented approach towards a patient-oriented approach.

1.1. Oncology Pharmacy-Definition and History

Since the concept of pharmaceutical care was introduced by Hepler and Strand in 1990, there have been significant changes in pharmacy practice worldwide (Hepler and Linda 1990). The first definition of pharmaceutical care was defined as "Pharmaceutical care is the responsible provision of drug therapy for the purpose of achieving definite outcome which improve patient quality of life." According to the definition, patient-centered services are the keystone of pharmaceutical care. These services include; curing of a disease, relieving patient's symptoms, slowing of a disease process and preventing a disease or symptoms. Recording patient data, assessment of DRPs, determination of therapeutic goal, determination of monitoring parameters, implementation of pharmaceutical care plan and monitorization of applicability of pharmaceutical care plan are the essential steps of pharmaceutical care. Pharmacists should have a "clinical pharmacy" education to give pharmaceutical care. According to the American College of Clinical Pharmacy (ACCP), "Clinical Pharmacy is a health science discipline in which pharmacists provide patient care that optimizes the drug therapy and promotes health, and disease prevention" (American College of Clinical Pharmacy 2020). This term has emerged from the traditional role of the pharmacist involving in the preparation, dispensing and selling of medications is no longer adequate and it leads to shift practice in pharmacy from drug product-centered to patient-centered, pharmaceutical care center.

Oncology pharmacist is a clinical pharmacist with have a special training in how to design, give, monitor, and change chemotherapy for cancer patients. Special training in oncology pharmacy has been available since the 1980s through residency or fellowship training programs (HOPA 2013). Nowadays OPs certificated by attending to the Board of Certified Oncology Pharmacist (BCOP) program. Both chemotherapeutic agents and supportive drugs have been used for the cancer treatment and this cause polypharmacy. The pharmacists are well positioned to provide the rational use and cost-effectiveness of various therapeutic options. Meanwhile, because of their positive contribution to oncology setting, pharmacists can increase the productivity of a medical care in practice. The OPs expanded roles can be evaluated under two main headings:

1. Responsibilities of preparation and administration of chemotherapeutics
2. Pharmaceutical care issues on oncology

1.2. Roles of OPs

1.2.1. Chemotherapy Preparation and Administration

The OPs are experts in drug therapy management, their responsibilities during chemotherapy preparation and administration are based on rational drug use and safe drug administration. OPs primary roles in oncology settings are as follows:

- Drug selection
- Drug supply
- Drug dispensing
- Dose adjustment
- Storage

- Compounding/dispensing
- Stability issues
- Safety use of medical devices
- Hazardous drug waste management
- Safe handling of chemotherapy

Most of chemotherapeutic agents are classificated as hazardous drugs. It is known that hazardous drugs have five serious characteristics that can be harmful to human. These hazardous effects are; genotoxicity, carcinogenicity, teratogenicity, fertility impairment/reproductive toxicity, serious organ toxicity at low doses. There have been many recent guidelines on safety handling of hazardous drugs published and revised every year by several organisations such as, National Institute for Occupational Safety and Health (NIOSH), American Society of Health System Pharmacists (ASHP), Occupational Safety and Health Administration (OSHA). OPs are the valuable information source for providing safe handling of chemotherapy drugs via educating the healthcare professionals and staffs according to these guidelines. Unfortunately, OPs can be faced some challenges on providing safety handling issues. Occasionally, problems may arise for health care personnel preparing chemotherapy medication to comply with personal protection measures. Also, the other staff, such as secretaries and employees working in the clinic may not be able to comply with these protection measures (using masks, wearing gloves etc.). OPs should encourage everyone in the clinic to take personal protection measures with continuing education and information. OPs should take adequate caution to prevent drug spills and inform personnel about potential risks of exposure and waste management.

Supply of closed system medical devices is another important issue that contributes positively on safe handling of chemotherapeutics. Sometimes there may be financial challenges which threaten hospitals supplies. Oncology pharmacists are valuable health professionals who can contribute to the selection of the most appropriate and economical medical devices for the preparation and application of chemotherapy drugs by following the developments in technology.

Compounding/dispensing and stability are very important issues since they are the last steps before the administration of chemotherapeutic drugs. Chemotherapy stability and preparation charts are available in most the of hospital settings. After the list of drugs prepared based on chemotherapy protocols frequently used in oncology clinics, OPs adds information on drug information labels (sometimes called stability charts) about the preparation of drugs and duration of stability by using reference sources (such as medicine information leaflets, medical databases).

One of the difficulties that oncology pharmacists frequently encounter in this process is the absence of stability data or variability of stability data in medicine information leaflets of different manufacturers. It is necessary to provide access to accurate and reliable information sources and to use these resources rationally for overcoming these problems in terms of patient safety and cost.

Oncology pharmacists play a key role in the preparation process of treatment protocols for patients. Chemotherapy treatment protocols determined under the leadership of organizations such as NCCN, ASCO, and ESMO and published in the most update manner. Many hospitals use the chemotherapy protocols frequently used in their oncology clinics. The chemotherapy treatment protocols contain information about, the dosage of drugs, the frequency of administration and the number of cycles that can be applied.

Pharmacists play an essential role in providing information on the correct preparation and administration of drugs included in the protocol. However, it is also the OPs responsibility to check the compliance of the planned protocol for the patient. Main difficulties that pharmacists may encounter during this process are as follows;

- Lack of Electronic Order System (manual records may contain spelling and number errors more often)
- Lack of adequate data of patient in order (weight, height, BSA, name-surname, identity number, name of the clinic)
- Presence of only total dose, lack of unit dose data (mg/m^2 and/or mg/kg)

- Presence of only total unit dose, lack of total dose data (mg/m^2 and/or mg/kg)
- Use of generic name instead of active ingredient name
- Lack of information about in which solution the drugs should be given
- Orders with the drugs prescribed in incompatible solutions

Since the OPs are responsible for the safe medication preparation, interprofessional communication and knowledge are the essential terms to overcome with challenges. OPs should follow these principles of the rational drug use and safe medication preparation and administration;

- Right patient
- Right medication
- Right dose
- Right time
- Right route
- Right documentation

Philips et al. (2001) reported that, the average of deaths due to the medication errors was 50,000 patients each year in the United States of America and medications errors with chemotherapeutic agents were the second-most common cause. In general, polypharmacy is seen in most of cancer treatments due to the use of combination of chemotherapy and supportive care drugs. Therefore, medication errors can be occurred during prescription, preparation, dispensing and administration process (Serrano-Fabiá et al. 2009, Ranchon et al. 2011, Jayanthi et al. 2016, Weiss et al. 2017, Uppugunduri et al. 2018). There are various studies on the frequency of medication errors in the inpatient and outpatient oncology settings (Walsh et al. 2009, Bruce et al. 2012). In a recent study Uppugunduri et al. (2018) have reviewed over 19,000 articles (published between 2000-2018 years) related to chemotherapy medication errors. This study demonstrated that, the highest number of chemotherapy medication errors were occurred during prescribing process (24.6%), and the other chemotherapy medication errors were occurred 0.50% in preparation, 0.03% in dispensing, and 0.02% to 0.10% in administering process, respectively. ASHP has published a guideline for preventing medication errors with chemotherapy and biotherapy in 2015 (Goldspiel et al. 2015). The guideline emphasizes that multidisciplinary monitoring of medication use and verification is needed for harmonization of medication error reporting. This guideline includes recommendations for healthcare organizations, prescribing systems and prescribers, pharmacists (preparation and dispensing), nurses (medication administration systems), patient education, manufacturers and regulatory agencies.

OPs have critical roles in providing safe preparation and administration of chemotherapeutic drugs and preventing medication errors. According to the ASHP guideline, healthcare organizations related to oncology, should establish committees with representatives from each discipline to develop policies and procedures for the safe drug use process. These policies and procedures should include educational and competency requirements for healthcare professionals and staffs. Education programs should include following topics:

1. Introduction to the chemotherapy drugs
2. Indications and uses
3. Routes of administration
4. Administration schedules
5. Dose adjustments (including overdose, cumulative dose, maximal dose that can be safely given during a single administration)
6. Storage conditions
7. Adverse effects
8. Drug interactions
9. Safe handling of hazardous drugs.
10. Strategies for rationale management of extravasation.

Although there are "oncology pharmacy" and "oncology nursing" certificate programs for pharmacists and nurses in most of the countries, the contents of these programs may not be the same and these certification programs may be absent in some countries. In addition to this, there are pharmacists working in most of the oncology clinics. One of the difficulties that pharmacists face during providing services in these clinics is the lack of adequate information. In recent years, these deficiencies are tried to be eliminated with courses and/or practical applications related to oncology pharmacy to undergraduate education and with the continuous training programs prepared by national health institutions for graduate pharmacists. The permanent solution to the problem is to review the educational content of the institutions at the undergraduate level, the content of the postgraduate certificate programs and the re-certification methods and making the necessary arrangements.

1.2.2. Pharmaceutical Care Issues on Oncology

Pharmaceutical care is a patient oriented approach rather than the drug or disease oriented approach. Oncology patients commonly face to multiple health problems beside cancer disease such as treatment related toxicities, comorbid diseases and treatment related adverse effects. Monitorization of comorbid diseases are as important as monitorization of cancer.

The anxiety, fear and sadness started with the diagnosis of cancer than replaced by the treatment's unwanted side effects. This situation negatively affects the quality of life of the patient and contributes negatively to the treatment compliance and ultimately the success of treatment. In many studies, it has been shown that oncology pharmacists in the multidisciplinary team contribute positively to the success of the treatment (Tezcan et al. 2017, Muluneh et al. 2018, Jackson et al. 2018, Sweiss et al. 2018, Whitman et al. 2018). Documentation should be done carefully and accurately during pharmaceutical care, otherwise, any deficiencies or inaccuracies in the data could adversely affect the pharmaceutical care process. Pharmaceutical care is a step- by-step process and should be prepared and applied in a patient-specific manner.

These steps are: Recording patient data, assessment of DRPs, determination of therapeutic goal, determination of monitoring parameters, implementation of pharmaceutical care plan and monitorization of applicability of pharmaceutical care plan.

The challenges that pharmacists may be faced during the implementation of the pharmaceutical care plan and the methods of management of these challenges will be discussed step-by-step.

a) *Recording patient data:* It is the most essential step for a viable patient-oriented pharmaceutical care. The sociodemographic information of the patient should be recorded completely. This information should include; patient id, name-surname, age, gender, height, weight, alcohol/cigarette use, drug allergy, type of cancer, chemotherapy protocols, history of surgery, other comorbid diseases, prescription and non-prescription medications (vitamins, birth control pills, herbs and dietary supplements). Laboratory parameters related to the patient's treatment and, if necessary, results of imaging studies should also be recorded. Finally, medical reports should be checked and recorded for easy insurance procedures. One of the difficulties experienced by pharmacists in this process is the difficulties in accessing patient data. Although electronic order systems have been started to be used, in many countries, each hospital often has its own data systems. Pharmacists may access some of the sociodemographic data of the patients, which have just been mentioned. Sometimes this information exists in the clinic and/or hospital archives in paper form only and not processed into data systems of the hospital; this makes it difficult for the pharmacist to access to the patient data. Medication reconciliation can be achieved by referring patients to the oncology pharmacist before the treatment. Medication reconciliation is the formal and standardized process of obtaining the full list of medications previously used by the patient. It is an important strategy for comparing the previous and the current drug regimen of patients. In addition it provides the safe use of medication via detecting, analysing and resolving the drug interactions in prescriptions (Vega et al. 2016). In many studies conducted on in- and out-oncology settings have shown that pharmacists-led medication reconciliation significantly decrease the medication errors (Weingart et al. 2007, Vega et al. 2016, Pulliam 2017, Phan et al. 2019).

Pharmacists should use a documentation system integrated with hospital databases which would be useful in recording patient files. There are publications suggesting that e-order systems largely prevent possible drug errors (Baker et al. 2008; Porterfield et. 2014; Lizano-Díez et al. 2014).

In conclusion, it will be useful to prepare standardized chemotherapy order forms with the collaboration of pharmacists, doctors and technicians and application of this form electronically. Additionally, the integration of electronic orders with hospital systems, and the approval of orders by both the doctor and the pharmacist, will greatly prevent possible errors.

    b) *Assessment of possible DRPs:* According to the Pharmaceutical Care Network Europe (PCNE), "A Drug-Related Problem is an event or circumstance involving drug therapy that actually or potentially interferes with desired health outcomes". The classification of DRPs has been done by PCNE, based on the definition. It is now available as a tool entitled "PCNE Classification for Drug-Related Problems V9.00" (Pharmaceutical Care Network Europe 2020). This tool consist three main domains which lead to identification and management of DRPs: problems, causes and interventions. This tool has been used in many studies for determining possible DRPs in oncology patients. (Abunahlah et al. 2018, Yokoyoma et al. 2018, Budiastuti et al. 2019, Umar et al. 2020). Frequently seen DRPs are; adverse drug reactions (ADRs), drug interactions, non-adherence, dose and dosage schedule.

In the process of determining DRPs, OPs communicate with patients and/or their relatives, doctors, nurses and other healthcare professionals. OPs identify, evaluate and analyse possible DRPs with the accurate information flow. Possible side effects, drug interactions and supportive treatment protocol are determined according to the appropriate treatment protocol planned for the patient. The difficulties encountered while identifying DRPs can be seen as; lack of access to accurate and reliable sources of information; lack of communication/accessibility with patients and/or patient relatives and deficiencies in communication with the multidisciplinary team. From the perspective of pharmacists; interdisciplinary professional programs, which include communication skills, should be organized and these programs should be mandatory. The continuing professional educations given with regular intervals would provide up-to-date information about cancer and supportive care treatment.

A "pharmaceutical care unit" should be established in each oncology clinic and cancer patients and relatives should be directed to this unit. Primary aim of this service is to provide a great convenience in determining the possible DRPs related to the treatment. Secondary aim of this service is to provide pharmaceutical care services, and also to provide a communication and contact point for healthcare professionals of the multidisciplinary team. The prevention of possible errors during the cancer treatment would be largely ensured by the cooperation between the patient and the multidisciplinary team.

c) *Determination of therapeutic goal:* The therapeutic goals in cancer treatment are curative and palliative. Multimodality therapies such as surgery, radiotherapy and drug therapies have been developed to achieve the therapeutic goals. While creating a pharmaceutical care plan the treatment goals are reviewed by the pharmacist and new treatment goals can be added. For example in case of a diabetic cancer patient, achieving normal blood glucose levels can be added as a new therapeutic goal. At this step, OPs require working in cooperation with both the patient and/or patient relatives and the multidisciplinary team for providing complete medication review. On the other hand, it is important to emphasize that pharmacists are the closest accessible health professionals for the patient and/or patient relatives. OPs should document all treatment goals and share with the multidisciplinary team.

It is known that medical treatment of cancer has many side effects. During pharmaceutical care, the treatment targets related to preventing and management of these side effects should be determined. In addition, other comorbid diseases such as diabetes and hypertension and treatment targets should be revised.

    d) *Determination of monitoring parameters:* Follow-up parameters should be established to evaluate the prognosis of the disease, to ensure the effectiveness of treatment and coping with the side effects. In addition, checking drug interactions, therapeutic drug monitoring (for the drugs with narrow therapeutic range), following levels of cancer markers and monitorization of comorbid diseases (hypertension, diabetes, hyperlipidaemia etc.) should be performed (Abunuhlah et al. 2018, Knezevic et al. 2020).

Important follow-up parameters for the evaluation of the prognosis of the disease are given in the guidelines. Cancer markers such as; carcinoembriogenic antigen, carbohydrate antigen 19-9 can be given as an example for these follow-up parameters. Imaging studies such as positron emission tomography (PET) and computed tomography are another important follow-up parameter for cancer prognosis. Evaluation and follow-up of these monitoring parameters are performed by oncologists. Pharmacists should educate the patients for the necessity of all these tests and control visits decided by the doctor. Some patients do not want to have these tests due to physical or psychological fatigue caused by cancer treatment and/or disease. One of the difficulties that pharmacists face is in persuading the patient for compliance. The patient should be explained why the tests are requested and how they are performed. Patient privacy should be considered during this training. For this reason training in a special room such as a pharmaceutical care unit would be appropriate.

Many cancer drugs have undesirable toxic effects such as; myelosuppression, alopecia, neurotoxicity, nephrotoxicity, nausea/ vomiting. These unwanted toxic effects can both decrease the patient's quality of life and cause to postpone of the treatment. Close monitoring is essential for the prevention, follow-up and management of side effects. Side effect monitoring parameters and desired tests may vary for different treatment protocols and drugs (Table 1). Performing and evaluating these tests before each treatment is important in order to determine the reversal of drug toxicity.

Table 1. Monitoring parameters for treatment-induced side effects

Chemotherapy protocol/drug name	Adverse drug reactions (Common)	Test
FOLFOX	Neuropathy Hand-foot syndrome Myelosupression	Physical examination CBC
Trastuzumab	Cardiotoxicity	ECG
Gemcitabine-Carboplatin	Myelosupression Nephrotoxicity Peripheral neuropathy	CBC BUN Cr Physical examination
Cisplatin-Etoposide	Myelosupression Nephrotoxicity	CBC BUN Cr
FOLFIRI+Bevacizumab	Myelosupression Proteinuria	CBC Urine analysis

FOLFOX: Folinic acid+fluorouracil+oxaliplatin; CBC: Complete blood count; ECG: Electrocardiogram; BUN: Blood urea nitrogen; Cr: Creatinin; FOLFIRI: Folinic acid+fluorouracil-irinotecan.

Drug interactions can be; a desired effect, an undesirable effect, or a parameter which requires monitoring. For example, when oxaliplatin-based chemotherapy is administered to a diabetic patient, blood glucose values should be monitored because oxaliplatin prepared in 5% dextrose solution and oxaliplatin can cause peripheral neuropathy. As an another example; If a nephrotoxic drug such as aminoglycoside is given to a patient receiving cisplatin-based chemotherapy, kidney function should be monitored. The record of the herbal products used by the patients should be kept completely. In patients receiving oral tyrosine kinase therapy, the toxicity of drugs should be monitored when using warfarin or another drug metabolised by cytochrome P450 enzyme systems.

Among the challenges faced by pharmacists during medication review:

- Failure to access to hospital system
- Lack of available complete patient medical history. Many cancer patients can have comorbid diseases. Cancer disease, chemotherapy and supportive medication may affect the prognosis of comorbid disease.
- Patients giving incomplete information and sometimes hiding information about use of medicines and/or herbal products.
- Since patients do not define over-the-counter (OTC) medicines and herbal products as medicines, they may not inform the pharmacist about use of these medicines. All prescription and non-prescription drug usage should be questioned while taking anamnesis.
- Lack of available database for checking drug-drug, drug-supplements, drug-herbal products and drug-food interactions
- Lack of monitorization of the side effects of cancer treatment

Patient education and patient follow-up are very important in this regard. The recorded information should be shared with the multidisciplinary team, and patients should be directed to the doctor for further examinations, if necessary.

e. *Implementation of pharmaceutical care plan:* The factors which cause difficulties for the OPs encounter during the implementation of the pharmaceutical care plan can be classified as;

1. Patient related
2. Healthcare professional related
3. Educational insufficient

OPs face these challenges while making and applying a pharmaceutical care plan for cancer patients (Okonta et al. 2012).

Patients may be exhausted due to the bureaucratic procedures associated with the diagnosis and treatment of cancer diseases and crowded hospitals. Patient may not want to be in contact with another health professional other than the doctor. From the pharmacist's perspective, this challenge can be resolved by informing patients about the responsibilities of OPs and enabling interviews with patients. As an easily accessible health professional OPs can work in collaboration with patient/patient relatives and as a health consultant provide pharmaceutical care service. A recent study Tezcan et al. (2017) investigated the pharmaceutical care service planned for colorectal cancer patients, demonstrated that approximately 50% of the interviews were started by patients who demand counselling from OPs.

Identifying and defining the responsibilities of pharmacists in the multidisciplinary team will largely eliminate the difficulties associated with other healthcare professionals. Rational drug use and patient safety are common goals for all healthcare professionals.

Education is one of the important issues to ensure the self-confidence of the pharmacist. Rational use of correct and reliable literature should be included in the educational content.

f. *Monitorization of applicability of pharmaceutical care plan:* The patients and pharmacist's collaboration and adherence to the planned pharmaceutical care service helps to resolve the potential/unexpected problems and provides success in reaching the therapeutic target. One of the challenged faced by the OPs is to ensure patient's adherence to the plan. Education performed by OPs increase the awareness of patients and institutional encouragement of the multidisciplinary team to comply with the patients' pharmaceutical plan will prevent the emergence of possible drug problems.

CONCLUSION

In European countries such as Germany, Denmark and Spain pharmaceutical care services for chronic diseases such as; hypertension, diabetes, asthma and heart diseases are supported by the governmental institutions (Barsteigiene et al. 2003, Herborg et al. 2007, Volmer et al. 2008, Waszyk-Nowaczyk et al. 2019, Kishimoto et al. 2020). There are many studies show that the pharmaceutical care plans prepared and applied specific to cancer patients that increase the success of treatment (Abunahlah et al. 2016, Tezcan et al. 2017; Yokoyoma et al. 2018; Umar et al. 2020). Considering the challenges of the pharmaceutical care services and coping methods; "The establishment of the pharmaceutical care units in the hospital, providing the accessibility of the units and informing the patient/patient relatives and other health personnel about the duties and responsibilities of oncology pharmacists will greatly contribute to the rational drug use and patient safety.

REFERENCES

Abunahlah, Nibal, Mesut Sancar, Faysal Dane, and Mustafa Kerem Özyavuz. 2016. "Impact of Adherence to Antiemetic Guidelines on the Incidence of Chemotherapy-Induced Nausea and Vomiting and Quality of Life." *International Journal of Clinical Pharmacy* 38 (6): 1464–76. doi:10.1007/s11096-016-0393-3.

Abunahlah, Nibal, Anfal Elawaisi, Fatih Mehmet Velibeyoglu, and Mesut Sancar. 2018. "Drug Related Problems Identified by Clinical Pharmacist at the Internal Medicine Ward in Turkey." *International Journal of Clinical Pharmacy* 40 (2): 360–67. doi:10.1007/s11096-017-0585-5.

American Cancer Society. 2019. "*Cancer Facts & Figures 2019.*" Accessed March 2020 https://www.cancer.org/research/cancer-facts-statistics/all-cancer-facts-figures/cancer-facts-figures-2019.html.

American College of Clinical Pharmacy. 2020. "*Definition of Clinicial Pharmacy.*" Accessed January 2020 https://www.accp.com/stunet/compass/definition.aspx.

Budiastuti, Rizky Farmasita, Maksum Radji, and Rini Purnamasari. 2019. "The Effectiveness of Clinical Pharmacist Intervention in Reducing Drug Related Problems of Childhood Acute Lymphoblastic Leukemia Patient in Tangerang District General Hospital, Indonesia." *Pharmaceutical Sciences and Research* 6 (1). doi:10.7454/psr.v6i1.3966.

Bruce, Katie, Laura Hall, Sarah Castelo, Misty Evans, and Haydar Frangoul. 2012. "Direct Provider Feedback To Decrease Chemotherapy Ordering Errors: The "Gray Envelope" Initiative". *Pediatric Blood & Cancer* 59 (7): 1330-1331. doi:10.1002/pbc.24224.

Goldspiel, Barry, James M. Hoffman, Niesha L. Griffith, Susan Goodin, Robert DeChristoforo, Capt Michael Montello, Judy L. Chase, Sylvia Bartel, and Jharana Tina Patel. 2015. "ASHP Guidelines On Preventing Medication Errors With Chemotherapy And Biotherapy". *American Journal of Health-System Pharmacy* 72 (8): e6-e35. doi:10.2146/sp150001.

Hepler, Charles D., and Linda M. Strand. 1990. "Opportunities and Responsibilities in Pharmaceutical Care." *American Journal of Health-System Pharmacy* 47 (3): 533–43. doi:10.1093/ajhp/47.3.533.

Herborg, Hanne, Ellen Westh Sørensen, and Bente Frøkjær. 2007. "Pharmaceutical Care in Community Pharmacies: Practice and Research in Denmark." *Annals of Pharmacotherapy* 41 (4): 681–89. doi:10.1345/aph.1h645.

HOPA. 2013. "*Scope of Hematology/Oncology Pharmacy Practice.*" Accessed January 2020 http://www.hoparx.org/images/hopa/resource-library/professional-tools/HOPA13_ScopeofPracticeBk.pdf;

Jackson, Kasey, Cathy Letton, Andy Maldonado, Andrew Bodiford, Amy Sion, Rebekah Hartwell, Anastasia Graham, Carolyn Bondarenka, and Lynn Uber. 2018. "A Pilot Study To Assess The Pharmacy Impact Of Implementing A Chemotherapy-Induced Nausea Or Vomiting Collaborative Disease Therapy Management In The Outpatient

Oncology Clinics." *Journal Of Oncology Pharmacy Practice* 25 (4): 847-854. doi:10.1177/1078155218765629.

Jayanthi, Mathaiyan, Tanvi, Jain, Biswajit, Dubashi, Gitanjali, Batmanabane. 2016. "Prescription, Transcription and Administration Errors in Out- Patient Day Care Unit of a Regional Cancer Centre in South India." *Asian Pacific Journal of Cancer Prevention* 17 (5): 2611-2617.

Knezevic, Claire E., and William Clarke. 2020. "Cancer Chemotherapy." *Therapeutic Drug Monitoring* 42 (1): 6–19. doi:10.1097/ftd.0000000000000701.

Kishimoto, Naomi, Mayuka Arimitsu, Yuki Iwane, and Yuka Kobayashi. 2019. "Provision of Pharmaceutical Summaries to Community Pharmacists by Hospital Pharmacists from an Acute Hospital." *Iryo Yakugaku (Japanese Journal of Pharmaceutical Health Care and Sciences)* 45 (2): 97–105. doi:10.5649/jjphcs.45.97.

Lizano-Díez, Irene, Pilar Modamio, Pilar López-Calahorra, Cecilia F Lastra, Jose L Segú, Antoni Gilabert-Perramon, and Eduardo L Mariño. 2014. "Evaluation of Electronic Prescription Implementation in Polymedicated Users of Catalonia, Spain: a Population-Based Longitudinal Study." *BMJ Open* 4 (11). doi:10.1136/bmjopen-2014-006177.

Muluneh, Benyam, Molly Schneider, Aimee Faso, Lindsey Amerine, Rowell Daniels, Brett Crisp, John Valgus, and Scott Savage. 2018. "Improved Adherence Rates and Clinical Outcomes of an Integrated, Closed-Loop, Pharmacist-Led Oral Chemotherapy Management Program." *Journal of Oncology Practice* 14 (6): e324-e334. doi:10.1200/jop.17.00039.

Okonta, Jegbefume Mathew et al.2012. "Barriers to Implementation of Pharmaceutical Care by Pharmacists in Nsukka and Enugu metropolis of Enugu State." *Journal of Basic and Clinical Pharmacy* 3 (2): 295-8. doi:10.4103/0976-0105.103823.

Phan, Ha, Macey Williams, Kelly Mcelroy, Bradley Burton, Denise Fu, and Anand Khandoobhai. 2019. "Implementation of a Student Pharmacist-Driven Medication History Service for Ambulatory Oncology Patients in a Large Academic Medical Center." *Journal of Oncology Pharmacy Practice* 25 (6): 1419–24. doi:10.1177/1078155219831066.

"Pharmaceutical Care Network Europe." 2020. Pharmaceutical Care Network Europe. Accessed March 23. https://www.pcne.org/.

Phillips, Jerry, Sammie Beam, Allen Brinker, Carol Holquist, Peter Honig, Laureen Y. Lee, and Carol Pamer. 2001. "Retrospective Analysis Of Mortalities Associated With Medication Errors". *American Journal Of Health-System Pharmacy* 58 (19): 1835-1841. doi:10.1093/ajhp/58.19.1835. (Phillips et al. 2001).

Porterfield, Amber, Kate Engelbert and Alberto Coustasse. "Electronic prescribing: improving the efficiency and accuracy of prescribing in the ambulatory care setting." *Perspectives In Health Information Management* 11 (2014): 1g.

Pulliam, Traci R. 2017. "Pediatric Hematology/Oncology Outpatient Care: the Effect of a Standardized Collaborative Medication Reconciliation Process." *Evidence-Based Practice Project Reports*. 105.

Ranchon, Florence, Gilles Salles, Hans-Martin Späth, Vérane Schwiertz, Nicolas Vantard, Stéphanie Parat, and Florence Broussais et al. 2011. "Chemotherapeutic Errors in Hospitalised Cancer Patients: Attributable Damage and Extra Costs." *BMC Cancer* 11 (1). doi:10.1186/1471-2407-11-478.

Serrano-Fabiá, Amparo, Asunción Albert-Marí, Daniel Almenar-Cubells, and N. Víctor Jiménez-Torres. 2009. "Multidisciplinary System For Detecting Medication Errors In Antineoplastic Chemotherapy." *Journal of Oncology Pharmacy Practice* 16 (2): 105-112. doi:10.1177/1078155209340482.

Siegel, Rebecca L., Kimberly D. Miller, and Ahmedin Jemal. 2019. "Cancer Statistics, 2019." *CA: A Cancer Journal for Clinicians* 69 (1): 7-34. doi:10.3322/caac.21551.

Shord Stacy S. and Medina Patrick J. 2014. "Cancer Treatment and Chemotherapy." In *Pharmacotherapy: A Pathophysiologic Approach*, edited by Joseph T. DiPiro, Robert L. Talbert, Gary C. Yee, Gary R. Matzke, Barbara G. Wells, L. Michael Posey, 4482-4571. New York: McGraw-Hill Education.

Sweiss, Karen, Scott M. Wirth, Lisa Sharp, Irene Park, Helen Sweiss, Damiano Rondelli, and Pritesh R. Patel. 2018. "Collaborative Physician-Pharmacist–Managed Multiple Myeloma Clinic Improves Guideline Adherence and Prevents Treatment Delays." *Journal Of Oncology Practice* 14 (11): e674-e682. doi:10.1200/jop.18.00085.

Tezcan, Songül, Fikret Vehbi Izzettin, Mesut Sancar, Nazım Serdar Turhal, and Perran Fulden Yumuk. 2017. "Role of Clinical Oncology Pharmacist in Determination of Pharmaceutical Care Needs in Patients with Colorectal Cancer." *European Journal of Hospital Pharmacy* 25 (e1). doi:10.1136/ejhpharm-2016-001188.

Umar, Rashida Muhammad, Sule Apikoglu-Rabus, and Perran Fulden Yumuk. 2020. "Significance of a Clinical Pharmacist-Led Comprehensive Medication Management Program for Hospitalized Oncology Patients." *International Journal of Clinical Pharmacy*. doi:10.1007/s11096-020-00992-8.

Uppugunduri, Chakradhara RaoS., Ramkumar Ashokkumar, Sureshkumar Srinivasamurthy, JanetJ Kelly, ScottC Howard, and Subramani Parasuraman. 2018. "Frequency of Chemotherapy Medication Errors: A Systematic Review." *Journal of Pharmacology and Pharmacotherapeutics* 9 (2): 86. doi:10.4103/jpp.jpp_61_18.

Vega, Triana González-Carrascosa, Jesús Francisco Sierra-Sánchez, María José Martínez-Bautista, Fátima García-Martín, Francisco Suárez-Carrascosa, and Jose Manuel Baena-Cañada. 2016. "Medication Reconciliation in Oncological Patients: A Randomized Clinical Trial." *Journal of Managed Care & Specialty Pharmacy* 22 (6): 734–40. doi:10.18553/jmcp.2016.15248.

Volmer, Daisy, Kaidi Vendla, Andre Vetka, J Simon Bell, and David Hamilton. 2008. "Pharmaceutical Care in Community Pharmacies: Practice and Research in Estonia." *Annals of Pharmacotherapy* 42 (7-8): 1104–11. doi:10.1345/aph.1k644.

Walsh, Kathleen E., Katherine S. Dodd, Kala Seetharaman, Douglas W. Roblin, Lisa J. Herrinton, Ann Von Worley, G. Naheed Usmani, David Baer, and Jerry H. Gurwitz. 2009. "Medication Errors Among Adults

And Children With Cancer In The Outpatient Setting." *Journal of Clinical Oncology* 27 (6): 891-896. doi:10.1200/jco.2008.18.6072.

Waszyk-Nowaczyk, Magdalena. 2019. "Implementation of Proffesional Pharmaceutical Counselling Scheme in Community Pharmacies In Poznan And Warsaw (Poland)." *Farmacia* 67 (3): 531–36. doi:10.31925/farmacia.2019.3.23.

Weingart, Saul N., Angela Cleary, Andrew Seger, Terry K. Eng, Mark Saadeh, Anne Gross, and Lawrence N. Shulman. 2007. "Medication Reconciliation in Ambulatory Oncology." *The Joint Commission Journal on Quality and Patient Safety* 33 (12): 750–57. doi:10.1016/s1553-7250(07)33090-0.

Weiss, Brian D., Melissa Scott, Kathleen Demmel, Uma R. Kotagal, John P. Perentesis, and Kathleen E. Walsh. 2017. "Significant and Sustained Reduction in Chemotherapy Errors through Improvement Science." *Journal of Oncology Practice* 13 (4): e329-e336. doi:10.1200/jop.2017.020842.

Whitman, Andrew, Kathlene DeGregory, Amy Morris, Supriya Mohile, and Erika Ramsdale. 2018. "Pharmacist-Led Medication Assessment And Deprescribing Intervention For Older Adults With Cancer And Polypharmacy: A Pilot Study." *Supportive Care in Cancer* 26 (12): 4105-4113. doi:10.1007/s00520-018-4281-3.

Yokoyama, Satoshi, Satoko Yajima, Akari Shimauchi, Chihiro Sakai, Shuji Yamashita, Yoshihiro Noguchi, Yoko Ino, Kazuhiro Iguchi, and Hitomi Teramachi. 2018. "Oncology Pharmacist Contributions to Treatment with Oral Anticancer Agents in a Japanese Community Pharmacy Setting." *Canadian Pharmacists Journal/Revue Des Pharmaciens Du Canada* 151 (6): 377–82. doi:10.1177/1715163518802865.

BIOGRAPHICAL SKETCH

Songül Tezcan

Affiliation: Assist. Prof. Dr.

Education:
- Ph.D. in Clinical Pharmacy Marmara University Faculty of Pharmacy 2010-2016
- Supervisor: Prof. Dr. Fikret Vehbi Izzettin
- PhD Thesis Title: Determination of Pharmaceutical Care Needs in Patients with Colon Cancer
- M.Sc. on Clinical Pharmacy Istanbul University 2006-2009
- Master Thesis Title: Investigating of Nephrotoxicity and Quality of Life in Patients Treated with Cisplatin Based Chemotherapy
- Supervisor: Prof. Dr. Fikret Vehbi Izzettin
- Bachelor on Pharmacy: Istanbul University Pharmacy Faculty 2006

Business Address: Marmara University Faculty of Pharmacy Clinical Pharmacy Department, Recep Tayyip Erdoğan Külliyesi, Başıbüyük Yolu, 34854 4/A, Başıbüyük/ Istanbul/Turkey

Research and Professional Experience:

Research Interest:
Improving pharmaceutical care and life quality in cancer patients, determination of new techniques for thereupatic drug monitoring, markers for diagnosis and follow up of cancer patients.

Teaching and Work Experience:
Assistant of Professor Marmara University Faculty of Pharmacy Clinical Pharmacy Department 2018-.. Research Assistant Marmara University Faculty of Pharmacy Clinical Pharmacy Department 2007-2017

- Led several seminars for undergraduate students
- Participate in several research projects
- Oncology Pharmacist in Marmara University School of Medicine Oncology Department Outpatient Chemotherapy Unit 2007-2015
- Supervisor Pharmacist at Chemotherapy Preparation Unit
- Responsible for pharmaceutical care of oncology patients

Professional Membership:
Society of Clinical Pharmacy – 2005-....
European Society of Clinical Pharmacy-2015-...

Publications:
1. Izzettin FV, Celik S, Acar RD, Tezcan S, Aksoy N, Bektay MY, Sancar M. The role of the clinical pharmacist in patient education and monitoring of patients under warfarin treatment. *J Res Pharm.* 2019; 23(6): 1157-1163.
2. Tezcan S, İzzettin FV, Sancar M, Turhal S, Yumuk PF. Role of clinical oncology pharmacist in determination of pharmaceutical care needs in patients with colorectal cancer *Eur J Hosp Pharm* Published Online First: 10 March 2017. doi: 10.1136/ejhpharm-2016-001188.
3. Altaie AH, Köseoğlu A, İzzettin FV, Sancar M, Tezcan S, Alqozbakr T, Aksu A. Observation Of Radiotherapy Related Acute Side Effects Occurrence and Management in Cancer Patients. *International Journal of Pharmacy.* 2016;6(2):11-19.
4. Tezcan S, Özdemir F, Turhal S, İzzettin FV (2013). *High performance liquid chromatographic determination of free cisplatin in different cancer types. der pharma chemica*, 2013; 5(5), 169-174., doi: 0975-413X.
5. Tezcan S, İzzettin FV, Sancar M, Yumuk PF, Turhal NS (2013). Nephrotoxicity Evaluation in Outpatients Treated with Cisplatin-Based Chemotherapy Using a Short Hydration Method. *Pharmacology and Pharmacy,* 2013;4(4), 296-302., Doi: 10.4236/pp.2013.43043).

6. Turhal NS, Dane F, Butur S, Kocak M, Telli F, Seber S, Kanitez M, Aktas B and Yumuk PF *'Efforts to Validate the Applicability of Established Chemotherapy Treatment in Turkish Cancer Patients'* Pharmaceutica, 2011;814-817.

Affiliations:
1. Tezcan S, Izzettin FV, Sancar M, Yumuk PF, Turhal S. Nephrotoxicity Evaluation in Outpatients Treated with Cisplatin-Based Chemotherapy Using a Short Hydration Method. *Pharmacology & Pharmacy*, 2013, 4, 296-302 (11 affiliations)
2. Tezcan S, Özdemir F, Turhal NS, İzzettin FV. High performance liquid chromatographic determination of free cisplatin in different cancer types. *Der Pharma Chemica*. 2013;5(5): 169-174. (8 affiliations)
3. Turhal NS, Dane F, Butur S, Kocak M, Telli F, Seber S, Kanitez M, Aktas B and Yumuk PF *'Efforts to Validate the Applicability of Established Chemotherapy Treatment in Turkish Cancer Patients'* Pharmaceutica, 2011;814-817 (1 affiliation)

Poster Presentations:
1. Tezcan Songül, Kizilkaya Melike, Sancar Mesut, İzzettin Fikret Vehbi (2018). Evaluation of knowledge and attitudes of patients and pharmacists on using herbal products. 47th ESCP Symposium on Clinical Pharmacy "Personalised Pharmacy Care" (Özet Bildiri/Poster) (Yayın No:4452956).
2. Kiliçaslan Özge, Sancar Mesut, Tezcan Songül, İzzettin Fikret Vehbi (2018). Evaluation of knowledge and attitudes of patients using eye drops/ointments.. *12th International Symposium on Pharmaceutical Sciences (ISOPS-12)*. (Özet Bildiri/Poster)(Yayın No:4452953)
3. İzzettin Fikret Vehbi, Tezcan Songül, Bingöl Özakpinar Özlem, Attallah Wafi, Yumuk Perran Fulden, Uras Fikriye (2017). Plasma Levels of Growth Arrest-Specific 6 in Colon Cancer Patients.

International Meeting on Education and Research in Health Sciences (IMER-HS) (Özet Bildiri/Poster)(Yayın No:3665328)

4. İzzettin FV, Tezcan S, Cakici G, Sahin Y, Sancar M. Evaluation of Pharmacists' Role Related to Corticosteroid Usage: Corticophobia. 46th ESCP Symposium on Clinical Pharmacy *"Science meets practice - towards evidence-based clinical pharmacy services,"* 9-11.10.2017;Heidelberg, Almanya.

5. Tezcan S, Tanir Gİ, Yilmaz H, Memiş S, Sahin Y, Yumuk PF, Rabus S. Assessment of chemotherapy-related educational needs of colorectal cancer patients. 46th ESCP Symposium on Clinical Pharmacy *"Science meets practice - towards evidence-based clinical pharmacy services"*, 9-11.10.2017;Heidelberg, Almanya. (poster sunuculuğu)

6. Tezcan S, Izzettin FV. Klinik Onkoloji Eczacılığı ve Farmasötik Bakım, 3. Uluslararası İlaç Ve Eczacılık Kongresi, 26-29 Nisan 2017, İstanbul, Türkiye. (poster sunuculuğu). [*Clinical Oncology Pharmacy and Pharmaceutical Care, 3rd International Congress on Drug and Pharmacy*, 26-29 April 2017, Istanbul, Turkey. (poster hosting).]

7. Şahin Y, Tezcan S. Bitkisel ürün-ilaç etkileşimlerinde eczacının rolü, 3. Uluslararası İlaç Ve Eczacılık Kongresi, 26-29 Nisan 2017, İstanbul, Türkiye. [*Herbal product-drug interactions role of the pharmacist, 3rd International Congress on Drug and Pharmacy*, 26-29 April 2017, Istanbul, Turkey.]

8. Işık M, Tanır Gİ, Tezcan S. Epidermal büyüme faktörü reseptörü inhibitörü ile ilişkili dermatolojik yan etkilerin yönetiminde klinik eczacının rolü. 3. Ulusal klinik eczacılık kongresi, 9-12 Şubat 2017, Antalya. [*The role of the clinical pharmacist in the management of dermatological side effects associated with epidermal growth factor receptor inhibitor*. 3. National clinical pharmacy congress, 9-12 February 2017, Antalya.]

9. Tezcan S, Torun B, Çakıcı G. Kortikosteroidlerin Kullanımına İlişkin Sorunların Çözümünde Klinik Eczacının Rolü. 3. Ulusal klinik eczacılık kongresi, 9-12 Şubat 2017, Antalya. [*The Role of*

the Clinical Pharmacist in the Solution of Problems Related to the Use of Corticosteroids. 3. National clinical pharmacy congress, 9-12 February 2017, Antalya].

10. Tezcan S, Köseoğlu A, AlTaie DH. Kanser tedavisinde onkoloji eczacısının rolü. 3. Ulusal klinik eczacılık kongresi, 9-12 Şubat 2017, Antalya (Çalıştay). [*The role of oncology pharmacist in cancer treatment*. 3. National clinical pharmacy congress, 9-12 February 2017, Antalya (Workshop).]

11. Sancar M, Apikoğlu-Rabuş Ş, Okuyan B, Tezcan S, Özkan Ö, Şahin Y, İzzettin FV, Küçükgüzel ŞG. Eczacılık Eğitiminde Klinik Uygulamaların Önemi: Marmara Üniversitesi Örneği, I. Ulusal Eczacılık Eğitimi ve Akreditasyon Kongresi, 9-10 Mayıs 2016, Ankara. [*The Importance of Clinical Practices in Pharmacy Education: The Case of Marmara University*, I. National Pharmacy Education and Accreditation Congress, 9-10 May 2016, Ankara.]

12. Tezcan Songül, Sancar Mesut, Turhal Serdar, Yumuk Perran Fulden, İzzettin Fikret Vehbi (2015). Kanser Hastalarında İlaç Kaynaklı Problemlerin Belirlenmesinde Klinik Onkoloji Eczacısının Rolü. 2. Uluslararası İlaç Ve Eczacılık Kongresi. [*The Role of Clinical Oncology Pharmacist in Identifying Drug Related Problems in Cancer Patients*. 2nd International Pharmaceuticals and Pharmacy Congress.]

13. D H, Altaie, Köseoğlu Aygül, İzzettin Fikret Vehbi, Tezcan Songül, Tayf Alqozbakr, Aksu A (2015). Observation of Dominant Occurance of Radiotherapy Related Acute Side Effects and Management. 44th *Escp Symposium*, 2015, Lisbon.

14. Tezcan Songül, İzzettin Fikret Vehbi, Sancar Mesut, Yumuk Perran Fulden, Turhal Serdar (2015). Determination of Pharmaceutical Care Needs in Patients with Colon Cancer at an Ambulatory Setting. 44th *Escp Symposium*, 2015, Lisbon.

15. Butur S, Ozdemir F, Izzettin FV. High- Performance Liquid Chromatographic Determination of Free Cisplatin in Plasma After Administration of Cisplatin. IMPPS-3 *Third International Meeting on Pharmacy&Pharmaceutical Sciences*, Istanbul, Turkey, 2010.

16. Tezcan S., İzzettin FV., Turhal S. "Evaluation of quality of life of patients' treated with cisplatin based chemotherapy." *40th ESCP Symposium on Clinical Pharmacy: Connecting Care & Outcomes*, Dublin, Ireland, 18-21-2011.
17. Konyalı T., Sancar M., Sarıca P., Tezcan S., Yesilyurt M., İzzettin FV., Attitude and use of herbal remedies among pregnant women. *41st ESCP Symposium on Clinical Pharmacy*, Barcelona, Spain, 29-31 October, 2012.
18. Butur S, İzzettin FV, Turhal S. Sisplatin İle Kombine Kemoterapi Uygulanan Hastaların Yaşam Kalitelerinin Değerlendirilmesi. IV. Ulusal Akciğer Kanseri Kongresi, Antalya. 10-14 Kasım 2010. [*Evaluation of the Quality of Life in Patients with CISPlatin combined chemotherapy*. IV. National Lung Cancer Congress, Antalya. November 10-14, 2010.]

Conferences Given (As Invited Speaker):
1. Tezcan S. Kanser Tedavisinde Klinik Eczacının Rolü. 3. Uluslararası İlaç Ve Eczacılık Kongresi, 26-29 Nisan 2017, İstanbul, Türkiye. [International Drug and Pharmaceutical Congress, 26-29 April 2017, Istanbul, Turkey].
2. Tezcan S. Kemoterapi İlaç Hazırlama Prensipleri. Kanser Tedavisinde Yan Etki Yönetimi Hemşirelik Sempozyumu, 22 Mart 2017, İstanbul. [Chemotherapy Drug Preparation Principles. Side Effect Management Nursing Symposium in Cancer Treatment, 22 March 2017, Istanbul].
3. Tezcan S. Kolon kanseri hastalarında farmasötik bakım. 3. Ulusal klinik eczacılık kongresi, 9-12 Şubat 2017, Antalya. [Pharmaceutical care in colon cancer patients. 3rd National Clinical Pharmacy Congress, 9-12 February 2017, Antalya].
4. Tezcan S. İlaç stabilitesi. 13. Türkiye Eczacılık Kongresi, 21-24 Aralık 2016, İstanbulTezcan S. 'Klinik Eczacılığın Bir Uzmanlık Alanı: Onkoloji Eczacılığı', 6.Klinik Eczacılık - Farmasötik Bakım Hızlandırılmış Semineri" 18-19-20 Mart 2011, Taksim-İstanbul. [Drug stability. 13. Turkey Pharmaceutical Congress, 21-24

December 2016, istanbultezc S. 'a Clinical Pharmacy Practice Areas: Oncology Pharmacy', 6.Klinik Pharmacy - Pharmaceutical Care Accelerated Seminar "18-19-20 December 2011, the Taksim-Istanbul].

Conferences and Courses Attended:
1. ESMO Course Essentials of Medical Oncology 1. Tıbbi Onkoloji Güncelleme Kursu, 26-30 November 2008, Istanbul.
2. İleri Klinik Araştırmacı Eğitim Programı, 27-28 Eylül 2012, İSTANBUL.
3. Marmara Üniversitesi Hayvan Deneyleri Yerel Etik Kurulu, 08-19/10/2012, İstanbul.
4. Ulusal Hasta Bilgilendirme Yarışması, 23-24 Nisan 2005, Ankara.
5. Ulusal Farmasötik Bakım ve Klinik Eczacılık Kongresi, 23-25 Eylül 2005, İstanbul.
6. Ulusal Hasta Bilgilendirme Yarışması, 23-24 Nisan 2007, Ankara.
7. İnterdisiplinerlik 2. Proje ve Araştırma Zirvesi, 09-10 Mayıs 2008, İstanbul.
8. 36th European Symposium on Clinical Pharmacy, Implementing Clinical Pharmacy in Community and Hospital Settings: Sharing Experience, 25-27 October 2007, Istanbul.
9. Yaşlanma ile İlgili Hastalıkların Moleküler Mekanizması ve Mikro Besinlerin Rolü Sempozyumu, 11 Eylül 2009, İstanbul.
10. Best of ASCO Annual Meeting' 11, 02 Haziran 2011, İstanbul.
11. Farmakogenetik ve Farmakogenomik Sempozyumu, 17 Ekim 2012, İstanbul.
12. 1.Ulusal Kamu Eczacıları Kongresi, 6-9 Aralık 2012, Antalya.

Projects:
1. 1003 Öncelikli Alanlar Ar Ge Projeleri Destekleme Programi, Tübitak Projesi, Araştırmacı: Tezcan Songül, Araştırmacı: Sancar Mesut, Yürütücü: Anlar Fatma Banu, 25/06/2014 (continued.) [1003 Priority Fields R&D Projects Support Program, Tübitak

Project, Researcher: Tezcan Songül, Researcher: Sancar Mesut, Coordinator: Anlar Fatma Banu, 25/06/2014 (continued.)].
2. Kolonkanseri Hastalarinda Farmasötik Bakim İhtiyaçlarinin Belirlenmesi, Yükseköğretim Kurumları tarafından destekli bilimsel araştırma projesi, Araştırmacı, 10/07/2013 - 14/03/2016 (ULUSAL). [Determination of Pharmaceutical Care Needs in Colon cancer Patients, Scientific research project supported by Higher Education Institutions, Researcher, 10/07/2013 - 14/03/2016 (NATIONAL)].

Professional Appointments: Honors:
- TUBİTAK-BİDEB 2209- Master of Science Scholarship- 2006
- TUBİTAK-BİDEB 2211 Doctorate Scholarship- 2010

Publications from the Last 3 Years:
1. Izzettin FV, Celik S, Acar RD, Tezcan S, Aksoy N, Bektay MY, Sancar M. The role of the clinical pharmacist in patient education and monitoring of patients under warfarin treatment. *J Res Pharm.* 2019; 23(6): 1157-1163.
2. Tezcan S, İzzettin FV, Sancar M, Turhal S, Yumuk PF. Role of clinical oncology pharmacist in determination of pharmaceutical care needs in patients with colorectal cancer *Eur J Hosp Pharm* Published Online First: 10 March 2017. doi: 10.1136/ejhpharm-2016-001188
3. Altaie AH, Köseoğlu A, İzzettin FV, Sancar M, Tezcan S, Alqozbakr T, Aksu A. Observation Of Radiotherapy Related Acute Side Effects Occurrence and Management in Cancer Patients. *International Journal of Pharmacy.* 2016;6(2):11-19.

In: Pharmacists
Editor: Line L. Villadsen

ISBN: 978-1-53618-018-3
© 2020 Nova Science Publishers, Inc.

Chapter 3

CURRENT CHALLENGES AND PERSPECTIVES OF PHARMACY IN MIDDLE EASTERN COUNTRIES

Hala Sacre[1,2], PharmD, Souheil Hallit[2,3],*, PhD, Aline Hajj[4], PhD and Pascale Salameh[2,5,6], PhD

[1]Drug Information Center, Order of Pharmacists of Lebanon, Beirut, Lebanon
[2]INSPECT-LB: Institut National de Sante Publique, Epidemiologie Clinique et Toxicologie, Beirut, Lebanon
[3]Faculty of Medicine and Medical Sciences, Holy Spirit University of Kaslik (USEK), Jounieh, Lebanon
[4]Laboratoire de Pharmacologie, Pharmacie Clinique et Contrôle de Qualité des Médicaments, Faculty of Pharmacy, Saint-Joseph University of Beirut, Beirut, Lebanon
[5]Faculty of Medicine, Lebanese University, Hadat, Lebanon
[6]Faculty of Pharmacy, Lebanese University, Hadat, Lebanon

---

* Corresponding Author's Email: souheilhallit@hotmail.com.

Abstract

Introduction: The pharmacy profession in the Middle East is facing several challenges with common features related to the system, education, and practice, as the vast majority of the population live in low- to middle-income countries.

Challenges: From an educational point of view, pharmacy suffers from several gaps: the use of classical teaching methods making little use of digital and active learning methods, the graduation of non-specialized pharmacists with a rare recognition of specialties, the non-application of quality standards in all institutions despite the presence of regional standards, and the dearth of research in pharmaceutical sciences. An additional major issue is the lack of coordination between pharmacy educational institutions and market labor stakeholders, leading to a mismatch between the learning outcomes, competencies and skills of new graduate pharmacists, and continuing professional development programs. Practice challenges consist mainly in shifting the perceived image of the pharmacist from a drug seller to a medication expert, by adopting the pharmacist's modern and internationally recognized roles ("The Nine-Star Pharmacist") and by including the clinical, ethical and research aspects of the profession in everyday practice. There is an oversupply of pharmacists in some countries, while other countries suffer from a deep need. The misdistribution of interprofessional tasks, the financial and administrative difficulties associated with the system, and the increased societal demand add to the complexity of pharmaceutical services offered by pharmacists in different sectors.

Perspectives: To overcome these challenges, pharmacists' associations in collaboration with stakeholders in the region, must develop appropriate strategic plans; it is also necessary that governmental and educational institutions recognize and consider specialized competencies and degrees, adopt and implement good pharmacy practice quality standards in community and hospital settings, and apply governance principles. The elaboration of core and specific competencies frameworks for different sectors of pharmacy would help bridging the gap between education and practice. Interprofessional education, collaboration, and communication are additional concepts to be applied in appropriate settings.

Keywords: challenges, education, Middle East, perspectives, pharmacy, practice, research

1. BACKGROUND

1.1. Health in Middle Eastern Countries

The Eastern Mediterranean region includes 22 countries: Afghanistan, Bahrain, Djibouti, Egypt, Iran, Iraq, Jordan, Kuwait, Lebanon, Libya, Morocco, Oman, Pakistan, Palestine, Qatar, Saudi Arabia, Somalia, Sudan, Syria, Tunisia, the United Arab Emirates, and Yemen. Except for Iran, Somalia, and Pakistan, all these countries are Arabic-speaking, thus considered to be Arab countries (Alsharif et al. 2019). From a cultural perspective, this region is mainly affected by Islam (90% of the population), and the vast majority of the population lives in low- to middle-income countries, with some exceptions (Gulf Cooperation Countries that are richer countries). Health care systems vary from a country to another, according to the country income and the size of the private versus public sector (Alsharif et al. 2019).

Historically, this region has seen improvements in life expectancy and other health indicators, even under stress. The armed conflicts, as well as population growth and ageing, are expected to significantly impact the region's health and resources (Mokdad et al. 2016). Nowadays, the burden of chronic diseases, such as diabetes, cardiovascular disease, and obesity is increasing, as is that of infectious diseases, poverty, population growth, the growing number of refugees, and other public health issues (Mokdad et al. 2014). Also, the current political situation will lead to deteriorated health conditions in the region and globally (Mokdad et al. 2016).

1.2. Pharmacy in Middle Eastern Countries

The density of pharmacists (measured as the number of pharmacists per 10,000 inhabitants) has increased between 2006 and 2012 in all World Health Organization (WHO) regions, including the Middle Eastern region (Bates et al. 2018). Up-to-date information on the number of graduates and practicing pharmacists is scarce. A study in 2008 found that at least 14,000 students (of whom more than 75% were from Egypt) were admitted yearly to the first year of pharmacy (5-year BS pharmacy program) (Kheir et al. 2008). In 2015, pharmacists' density to population ranged between 17.5/10.000 in Lebanon, 13.5/10.000 in Jordan, and 0.1/10.000 in Morocco and Somalia, showing oversupply in some countries and a deep need in others (Alsharif et al. 2019). In Saudi Arabia, the distribution of pharmacists is inequitable between native and immigrants (Almaghaslah et al. 2019), highlighting the need to better train Saudi citizens as pharmacists (AlRuthia et al. 2019).

Nevertheless, an increased number of available pharmacists does not necessarily mean an improved quality of pharmaceutical care. In fact, at the international level, the WHO and the International Pharmaceutical Federation (FIP) have jointly identified new roles for pharmacists through the "Nine-Star pharmacist" that represents the modern and skilled pharmacist, educated to have the required competencies and apply patient-centered care (Thamby SA and Parasuraman S 2015). This concept, introduced in 2007, represents a challenge to be implemented in the region, where pharmacy is still practiced in a relatively old way, and the number of credentialed pharmacists per country (with a Board of Pharmacy Specialties) are very low compared with non-specialized pharmacists (Alsharif et al. 2019). Currently, some pharmacists might also hold a PharmD (6-year program) at entry-level, instead of the traditional 5-year BS degree, which should theoretically add to their clinical skills and be expected to improve pharmaceutical services in all sectors (Alsharif et al. 2019). Nevertheless, advances in pharmacy education have a different pace in the region, and even when changes are relatively rapid, those of pharmacy practice appear to be slower (Kheir et al. 2008).

Although the pharmacy profession is steadily evolving (Kheir N 2013) and despite identifying new roles for the pharmacist (Thamby SA and Parasuraman S 2015), in the Middle Eastern region, pharmacy is still lagging behind the rest of the world. Several factors are limiting the pharmacist to the routine of dispensing medications, which explains why most pharmacists work in the community setting (most community pharmacies being privately owned). In some countries such as the Kingdom of Saudi Arabia, where permitted by law, chain pharmacies started to show growth, particularly in urban areas and malls, but in most places, they have not taken over the majority of pharmacies (Kheir N 2013). As in other parts of the world, hospital pharmacy practice is generally more advanced than community practice, and pharmacists working in hospital settings are more likely to have advanced degrees or residency training (Al-Ghananeem et al. 2018). As for the industrial sector, many regional countries have a robust pharmaceutical industry, with more than 200 pharmaceutical manufacturers located in the Arab world and global pharmaceutical sales of 2% in the Middle East and North Africa (MENA) region, making this sector an influential stakeholder in the pharmacy profession (Al-Shareef et al. 2016).

Consequently, pharmacy in the Middle East (ME) might be evolving slowly and differently, with relatively little information available in the English press. Overall, it is facing several challenges with common features related to education, research, and practice.

2. CHALLENGES RELATED TO PHARMACY EDUCATION

From an educational point of view, pharmacy suffers from several gaps.

2.1. Failure to Apply Quality Standards

All universities teaching pharmacy have a national certification from competent authorities, but no country in the region has established national quality standards yet, except for the GCC countries where general, not pharmacy-related, standards are in the development phase. Although all universities teaching pharmacy are nationally certified, very few have international accreditation from recognized pharmacy authorities (Alkhateeb et al. 2018, Alsharif et al. 2019). This seems related to several challenges, including socioeconomic and political instability, limited obligation to implement accreditation and quality assurance, insufficient engagement of professional organizations, disconnection between academia, practice, and regulatory sectors, curricula shortcomings, skills gaps, absence of competency frameworks, inconsistencies in the processes of pre-registration, training, and professional development (Bajis et al. 2018). Also, many countries face significant cultural, logistical, and legal barriers to accreditation, and lack design studies for a consensual approach to this process, including quality standards, basic skills and specific, educational outcomes and programs (Al-Ghananeem et al. 2018).

2.2. Lack of Coordination with Market Labor Stakeholders

The lack of coordination between pharmacy educational institutions and market labor stakeholders during curricular engineering leads to a mismatch between the learning outcomes, competencies, and skills of new graduate and specialized pharmacists. The design of curricula should use modern methods, including competencies needed in the labor market, and gaps assessed during practice (Bajis et al. 2016), as well as the motivations, and learning/career aspirations of students (Awad, Al-Haqan, and Moreau 2017). However, frustration is echoed throughout the region about the disparity or "gap" between what is taught in theory and the extent to which it is applied in real practice settings (Bajis et al. 2016). Consequently, the lack of standardization is leading to the graduation of pharmacists with heterogeneous skills at entry-level.

In addition, most universities offering pharmacy degrees, whether BS Pharm or PharmD, do not offer post-graduate education programs (master's degree or residency training), thus resulting in a vast majority of unspecialized pharmacy graduates in the region (Al-Qadheeb et al. 2012). Furthermore, in some countries like Lebanon, where pharmacy specialties are still not recognized, pharmacists are discouraged from pursuing higher education (Sacre, Tawil, Hallit, Hajj, et al. 2019, Sacre, Tawil, Hallit, Sili, et al. 2019), thus resulting in large numbers of non-specialized pharmacists, with few practice positions filled out by pharmacists with appropriate skills at entry-level, as fresh graduates would need additional trainings and a long experience to be able to practice in an optimal way. In addition, sometimes the situation may be reversed: the few specialized pharmacists might be considered overqualified for some positions and consequently underpaid, further discouraging other pharmacists from specializing. These factors further translate into a profound mismatch with the labor market needs of highly specialized professionals in several practice fields (Sacre, Hallit, et al. 2019).

2.3. Traditional Teaching Methods

Making little use of digital and active learning methods while favoring traditional teaching methods could undervalue the expected outcomes. In the Middle East, only half of the teachers in health professions, including pharmacy, use active learning; the most commonly cited barriers to implementing active learning were time constraints and lack of technical support (AlRuthia et al. 2019). Some countries, such as Qatar, have started to apply modern teaching techniques, such as blended learning, and have found highly satisfactory results, but not without obstacles to overcome (Wilbur and Taylor 2018). A Qatari university also tested Problem Based Learning (PBL) and tackled strengths (novelty, improved learning, engagement, and alignment with accreditation), weaknesses (student preparation and buy in, inconsistent facilitation, and logistical support), opportunities (expansion, departmental support, timing, and congruence with practice skills), and challenges (student resistance, departmental engagement, assessment, expansion, and cultural norms in teaching and learning) (Nasr and Wilby 2017). The use of active pedagogic strategies in Saudi Arabia, such as self-reflection and peer-assessment, significantly improved examination performance, facilitated deep and constructive engagement with learning and fostered students' confidence in the use of critical thinking and clinical decision-making (Yusuff 2015). In Iraq, in the absence of university emails, the use of Facebook improved the communication between faculty members and students (Al-Jumaili, Al-Rekabi, Alsawad, et al. 2017). It is worth noting that in the current COVID-19 crisis, several universities of the ME are starting to establish distance learning using digital methods; further studies will be necessary to assess the effectiveness of such measures with some resistance among teachers and students, due to unpreparedness and internet connections instability in some regions (personal communication with teachers form Lebanon, Syria, and the United Arab Emirates).

2.4. Inadequacy of Assessment and Evaluation Methods

Despite their demonstrated importance in improving the pharmacy education system, assessment and evaluation methods are still not fully modernized in the region. Some universities started applying newer methods, such as the Objective Structured Clinical Examination (OSCE), which had acceptable validity and reliability, but not without difficulties (assessment tools, standardized actors, assessor calibration, and standard setting) (Wilby and Diab 2016, Sobh et al. 2017). A useful assessment framework was also suggested to coordinate assessment plans and support the quality of programs; it consisted of three domains: programmatic assessment, academics, and engagement/satisfaction (Wilby et al. 2017).

2.5. Difficulties in Adapting Experiential Education to Required Competencies

Some universities have difficulties in correctly adapting experiential education (trainings) to required competencies. This might be due to students' unpreparedness and experiential settings used despite being inappropriate (inadequate equipment, unavailability of preceptors, remote regions, etc.). Essential measures are generally recommended to improve trainings, such as effective communication between the university, preceptors, and students, scheduled site visits, fair wages and compensation for preceptors, financial support for training sites, preparatory workshops for the students, and non-clinical rotations (Sales et al. 2019). In some cases, community pharmacy preceptors needed additional skills, such as in Qatar, where they showed poor knowledge and understanding of evidence-based medicine, an essential component in precepting pharmacy students. Thus, it was recommended to adapt the curriculum accordingly to instill this concept to future pharmacists (Paravattil, El Sakrmy, and Shaar 2018).

2.6. Gaps in Knowledge in Specific Topics, Populations, and Situations

Gaps in the curricula might be identified before or after graduation by assessing the knowledge of practicing pharmacists. In addition to standard curricula, there is a need to add or elaborate courses related to specific topics, populations, or situations in the region. Practicing Qatari pharmacists reported the need to enhance infectious disease content in the curriculum and close gaps related to microbial stewardship trainings (Nasr, Higazy, and Wilbur 2019). Also, in the United Arab Emirates, university students' knowledge about antibiotics, including pharmacy students, indicated a gap in curricula (Jairoun et al. 2019). Other areas with gaps in knowledge include but are not limited to, geriatrics (Zolezzi et al. 2018), complementary and alternative medicine (Radi et al. 2018), nanotechnologies (Assali et al. 2018), generics' substitution (Shraim et al. 2017, Al-Tamimi et al. 2016, Alrasheedy et al. 2014), and clinical pharmacokinetics (Kheir et al. 2015), or pharmacogenomics (Elewa et al. 2015).

2.7. Scarcity of Interprofessional Education (IPE)

Inter-professional education (IPE) has demonstrated its efficacy in developed countries. Thus, pharmacy academics across the Middle East have shown their readiness to implement it in their educational settings. However, the barriers that impeded its implementation in health professions included cultural challenges, scheduling shared courses and activities, in addition to limited resources (El-Awaisi et al. 2016). Further challenges might also include burdened curriculum, leadership, stereotypes and attitudes, diversity of students, designing IPE, teaching, enthusiasm, professional jargon and accreditation, assessment of learning, as well as security and logistics issues (Farra et al. 2018).

2.8. Continuing Professional Education and Development Programs

As with other medical sciences, pharmaceutical sciences are continually evolving worldwide, making it difficult for pharmacists to stay current. The volume of pharmaceutical literature is on the increase, and it is vital to use appropriate resources to optimize patients' therapeutic outcomes. Thus, continuing education and professional development are required to offer the most appropriate pharmaceutical care to patients. In the Middle Eastern region, several studies show that the knowledge of pharmacists is not optimal. In Iraq, professional knowledge and pharmaceutical care are major concerns (Abdulameer 2018). A similar lack of knowledge on the application of evidence-based medicine in real-life practice was reported in Kuwait (Buabbas et al. 2018). On the other hand, practicing pharmacists might be reluctant to enroll in continuing education programs; reasons cited include mainly work and family obligations, lack of interest, lack of time, lack of value and motivation, commuting difficulties, computer illiteracy, and difficulty using technology (Sacre, Tawil, Hallit, Sili, et al. 2019, Sacre, Tawil, Hallit, Hajj, et al. 2019).

Nowadays, health technology and computer literacy are considered a necessity closely linked to professional development: contemporary pharmacy-related activities and programs require the pharmacist to be knowledgeable about computers, which is not always the case in Middle Eastern countries. For example, in Lebanon, although using electronic applications was shown to be useful to screen for non-communicable diseases among underserved populations (Saleh et al. 2018), pharmacists in remote regions may not have internet access or any connected device (Sacre, Tawil, Hallit, Hajj, et al. 2019).

3. CHALLENGES RELATED TO PHARMACY RESEARCH

Although one of the roles of pharmacists is to conduct research (Sam and Parasuraman 2015), research related to pharmacy is rare in the Middle East, in comparison with the Western world. Collaborative projects between teams from the region are rare, while collaborations with developed countries might be more common. There is also a need to improve the quality and reporting of studies from Middle Eastern countries. The reasons for the dearth of pharmaceutical research in the region might include:

3.1. Lack of Research Strategies at Institutional, National and Regional Levels

Although few institutions and countries have worked on establishing a clear research agenda or strategy, such as Iran (Mansoori et al. 2018) and Qatar (Elkassem et al. 2013), this point remains to be better established at the national and regional levels.

3.2. Lack of Exposure to Research during Pre-Graduate Years

Students not being exposed to research leads to the underestimation of research importance by practicing pharmacists and their lack of involvement in research (except for those in academic settings) (Elkassem et al. 2013), although pharmacists are sometimes interested in getting involved in research (Zeidan, Hallit, et al. 2019). Due to noticed gaps regarding research knowledge among graduates, universities need to include research related courses and topics in their bachelors' program curriculum, in order to make pharmacists equipped in terms of research knowledge, regardless of the career path they choose (Mukattash et al. 2017). More in-depth research education can be applied, based on specific competencies, to promote the contribution of pharmacists to research after graduation (Hallit, Hajj, Sacre, et al. 2019). A better knowledge about Evidence Based Medicine is also needed, because it affects decision making during practice (Abu Farha et al. 2014).

3.3. Lack of Adequate Resources Related to Working Positions, Funds and Skills

There is a lack of positions for researchers-pharmacists in the region: even in the academic sector, pharmacists with research credentials are hired and expected to teach and serve, while research is rarely mandatory or adequately valued in teaching institutions (Hallit, Hajj, Sacre, et al. 2019). Moreover, although a minority of pharmacists are involved in basic, experimental or observational research projects, methods are not always optimal, most probably due to finances or skills insufficiency (Nazer et al. 2018, Stewart et al. 2015). Strategies to improve the quality of future studies in several fields are required, such as in health economics and pharmacoeconomics, since there is a deficiency in the quality of articles, in performing a full economic evaluation and choosing societal perspective (Eljilany et al. 2018). Another example is using standardized approaches to quantify medication errors' prevalence, severity, outcomes and contributory factors is also warranted in Middle Eastern countries (Thomas et al. 2019).

3.4. Lack of Advanced, Experimental and Translational Research

Although academic research projects focusing on simple basic sciences and observational research stemming from clinical aspects of pharmacy are common, advanced experimental clinical trials and translational research are not well developed in the region. The professional aspects of pharmacy practice also remain to be further researched (Elkassem et al. 2013).

The majority of published research is related to observational studies, such as polymedication consequences (Naser et al. 2018, Huang et al. 2018), medication errors causes (Stewart, Thomas, MacLure, Pallivalapila, et al. 2018, Al Juffali et al. 2019), post-marketing comparison of drug classes (Almalag et al. 2018), or also generating/validating scales for diagnosing/screening diseases and following up treatments (Alsous et al. 2017, Hallit, Raherison, Malaeb, et al. 2019, Hallit et al. 2018, Shilbayeh, Alyahya, et al. 2018, Zakaria et al. 2018, Hallit, Sacre, Haddad, et al. 2019, Mourad et al. 2019, Zeidan, Haddad, et al. 2019, Saade et al. 2019, Haddad et al. 2019, Hallit, Raherison, Waked, et al. 2019, Hallit, Raherison, et al. 2017), and medication use (Ayoub, Musalam, and Abu Mahadi 2017, Shilbayeh, Almutairi, et al. 2018).

4. CHALLENGES RELATED TO PHARMACY PRACTICE

Practice challenges consist mainly in shifting the perceived image of the pharmacist from a drug seller to a medication expert, by adopting the pharmacist's modern and internationally recognized roles - "The Nine-Star Pharmacist," as stated above (Thamby SA and Parasuraman S 2015) - and by including the clinical, ethical and research aspects of the profession in everyday practice. Calls to action have been reported by several stakeholders (academics, professionals and authorities), but challenges are numerous, related to specificities of the context, rapid changes of the profession itself worldwide, and low capacities of systems to adapt to difficulties. Pharmaceutical services offered by pharmacists in different sectors are complex, and challenges related to pharmacy practice include:

4.1. Financial and Administrative Difficulties Associated with the System

Pharmacists in the community might have financial difficulties in some Middle Eastern countries, leading to understaffing, overwhelming professional stress (Hallit, Zeenny, et al. 2017) and work fatigue (Sacre, Obeid, et al. 2019). In fact, these difficulties might be linked to the healthcare system structure and processes that are not adapted yet to the new business models adopted in western countries, where pharmacists' services are remunerated separately from the medication prices. Even in countries where pharmacy practice is relatively advanced, there are still challenges of this type that hamper appropriate performance of pharmacists: in a study on medication safety culture in Jordan, "understaffing, work pressure, and pace" were reported as major weaknesses, and pharmacists pointed the need for adequate breaks between shifts, and a less distractible work environment to perform their jobs accurately (Alsaleh et al. 2018). In Qatar, stress, workload and lack of staff at key times were perceived to be major contributors to medication errors, affecting patient safety (Stewart, Thomas, MacLure, Pallivalapila, et al. 2018). In the UAE, restrictive legislations, negative public perception, lack of time and support staff were considered barriers to delivering professional services (Alzubaidi, Saidawi, and Mc Namara 2018). In Lebanon, cited barriers to the provision of medication therapy management were inadequate time, workflow and physical space (Domiati et al. 2018). Such a gap in health systems of low- and middle-income countries was demonstrated at the levels of oversight, funding, and infrastructure supporting health services caring for patients (Bello et al. 2018).

4.2. Dissatisfaction and Mental Health Issues of Pharmacists

The satisfaction and mental health of pharmacists seems to be affected by professional difficulties and stress; this aspect was studied in several Middle Eastern countries. In Lebanon, community pharmacists have high levels of stress, mental and physical work fatigue, insomnia and depression (Sacre, Obeid, et al. 2019). Similarly, low levels of job-related satisfaction were found for pharmacists in Iran (Moghadam et al. 2014). In Jordan, community pharmacists were found to be less satisfied with their jobs than their hospital counterparts. Pharmacists' job satisfaction should be enhanced to improve pharmacists' motivation and competence. Consequently, this will improve their productivity and provision of pharmaceutical care (Al Khalidi and Wazaify 2013).

4.3. Misdistribution of Interprofessional Tasks and Harmful Stereotypes

In the region, there is a clear lack of collaborative practice, in addition to hierarchy and power play between health professionals (El-Awaisi et al. 2018). Exploration of collaboration/communication between pharmacists and physicians in the practice fields are ongoing. In Iran, although declared opinion about physician-pharmacist' collaboration was positive, it did not match the real experience (Alipour, Peiravian, and Mehralian 2018). Barriers arising are numerous, such as patient and physician acceptance, logistic and financial issues and perceived pharmacist competence as declared in the United Arab Emirates (Hasan et al. 2018). In Iraqi hospitals, physician-pharmacist collaboration was positively affected by the role specification and relationship initiation for physicians, and the role specification and trustworthiness for pharmacists (mainly academic affiliation) (Al-Jumaili, Al-Rekabi, Doucette, et al. 2017). We note that the lack of collaboration with physicians, added to the deficient quality of prescription writing are increasing the risk of medication errors (Kamel et al. 2018, Al-Worafi et al. 2018).

4.4. Patients Erroneous Perceptions and Behaviors

In general, the Middle Eastern countries populations have low to moderate health literacy (Abdel-Latif and Saad 2019), and wrong beliefs towards medications (Alhaddad et al. 2014). A study in Lebanon showed suboptimal medication-related knowledge among patients, and suboptimal patient's interactions with their primary care givers (Ramia et al. 2017). In Saudi Arabia, prescription label misunderstanding was common among elderly, lower socioeconomic status and less educated patients (Alburikan et al. 2018). Other erroneous perceptions lead to the misuse of certain medications, such as antibiotics; inappropriate drug use such as wrong indication, short and long duration of treatment, sharing and storing antibiotics at home for future use are common (Alhomoud et al. 2017). Difficulty accessing healthcare services, participant's cultural beliefs and practices, erroneous perceptions of antibiotics efficacy and knowledge about antibiotic resistance are among cited reasons (Alhomoud, Aljamea, and Basalelah 2018).

4.5. Over-the-Counter Availability of a Wide Range of Medications

One major challenge pharmacists face/contribute to in the region is the delivery of medications without prescription; pharmacists should either be ready for this endeavor or refrain from it to avoid its deleterious consequences (Hijazi et al. 2016), given particularly that some of these practices are illegal in several countries (Yaacoub et al. 2019). In a systematic review about medications misused in the Middle East, involved products included: codeine containing products, topical anesthetics, topical corticosteroids, antimalarial, and of course, antibiotics (Khalifeh, Moore, and Salameh 2017).

Reasons for over-the-counter use include the ease of access to community pharmacies compared to other healthcare services, claimed expertise and knowledge of pharmacists and patients' trust, misconceptions and inappropriate practices of the public towards antibiotic use, customer pressure, pharmacists' need to ensure business survival and weak regulatory enforcement mechanisms (Alhomoud, Almahasnah, and Alhomoud 2018). Patients' attitude towards the disease and the physician, unfriendly environments, influence of others, were also reasons cited for self-medication among elderly in Iran (Mortazavi et al. 2017). Other reasons include poor national medicines regulations, limited availability of qualified pharmacists, commercial pressure on pharmacy staff, consumer demand, inappropriate prescribing practices and lack of awareness of resistance

(Sakeena, Bennett, and McLachlan 2018). Moreover, pharmacists, friends, or parents were found to be the main sources of medication misuse all over the region (Khalifeh, Moore, and Salameh 2017). For some substances, there is even a potential for abuse, the problem having a large prevalence in Middle Eastern countries, such as Saudi Arabia (Ibrahim et al. 2018), and Yemen (Abood and Wazaify 2016).

4.6. Increased Societal Demand on Pharmacists and Pharmaceutical Care in Challenging Conditions

Pharmaceutical care plays a crucial role in optimizing medication use and improving patient outcomes, whilst preventing medication misuse and reducing costs. Evidence also suggests that pharmacists' counselling improves clinical outcomes, quality of life, drug and disease knowledge and reduces health service utilization. Given the pharmacists' accessibility, patients rely on them to participate in clinical services (Iskandar et al. 2017), and give advice on clinically complex questions, which is not always happening (Awad, Al-Rasheedi, and Lemay 2017, Alaqeel and Abanmy 2015). The lack of appropriate skills, regulations and environment are major barriers to pharmaceutical care implementation (Mehralian et al. 2014).

Nevertheless, pharmacists should be ready from viewpoints of knowledge (appropriate information delivery), attitude (courtesy and respect) and competency (communication and trustworthiness) to satisfy the patients (Mehralian, Rangchian, and Rasekh 2014, Iskandar et al. 2017). Patients' trust in their pharmacists might especially be affected by perception of pharmacist communication and technical competence (Siddiqua et al. 2018).

Examples of important pharmaceutical services in the community include advice on contraception (El-Mowafi and Foster 2019), vaccination (Alshammari, Yusuff, et al. 2019, Gamaoun 2018), headache (Hammad et al. 2018), specific Middle eastern diseases such as MERS-CoV (Aldohyan et al. 2019), special populations' care such as children (Mukattash et al. 2018), elderly (Ertuna et al. 2019, Aljadani and Aseeri 2018), pregnant

(Rouf et al. 2018) or breastfeeding women (Albassam and Awad 2018, Abduelkarem and Mustafa 2017), and special situations such as Ramadan fasting issues among diabetics (Alluqmani et al. 2019) or in case of medication errors (Karimian et al. 2018, Abu Farha et al. 2018). Additional services are also required in the hospitals, such as the participation to antimicrobial stewardship and accreditation activities (Alghamdi et al. 2018).

4.7. Medication Adherence Issues among Patients

Middle Eastern patients have adherence issues with medications; the problem was reported in several countries (Jaam et al. 2017). Barriers to medication adherence included: 1) patient-related factors, which included patients' individual characteristics and patients' perception, attitude and behavior; 2) patient-provider factors, which included communication and having multiple health care providers caring for the patient; and 3) societal and environmental factors, which included social pressure and traveling to visit friends and relatives. The intervention of pharmacists is of major importance to improve patients' adherence. Examples include Qatar (Jaam et al. 2018), Kuwait (Lemay, Waheedi, et al. 2018), and Lebanon (Fahs et al. 2018), since patients with better adherence are known to have better outcomes, especially for chronic diseases (Haddad et al. 2018).

4.8. Extended Duties of Community Pharmacists

In some countries, authorities may rely on pharmacists' contribution to public health promotional activities and programs, such as providing education to stop tobacco chewing, smoking, alcohol drinking and improve oral hygiene in Yemen (Yousuf et al. 2019), or in Qatar (El Hajj et al. 2019). In some countries, pharmacists need to conduct medication use reviews (MUR), a role to which they do not seem to be sufficiently ready (Babiker, Carson, and Awaisu 2014).

4.9. Counterfeit and Suboptimal Medications on the Market

Although not always quantified, the region's developing countries have a significant percentage of counterfeit and suboptimal medications. The topic being sensitive, very few data is available regarding the healthcare professionals (including pharmacists) and the general population knowledge and attitude about this issue. In Lebanon, some researchers found the need for additional awareness campaigns with an emphasis on the role that pharmacists have in protecting patients from using counterfeit medications. In addition, a need for an official definition that distinguishes between the different types of counterfeiting has been noted (Sholy et al. 2018).

As for suboptimal medications, they are also available in the region to reduce health related cost; however, since some generics with suboptimal manufacture might be marketed without proper testing (Hobeika et al. 2020): physicians prescribe them, pharmacists deliver them and patients suffer of their inadvertent related consequences if inappropriately used. Although progress has been made with regards to enhancing generic substitution in some countries such as Lebanon and Saudi Arabia, it remains important to educate patients about generic medicines and plan context-specific schemes that promote prescribing and dispensing of generic drugs among physicians and pharmacists (Saleh et al. 2017, Alkhuzaee et al. 2016, El-Jardali et al. 2017).

4.10. Underreporting of Adverse Events and Medication Errors

Adverse events related to drugs are common in the region, causing significant morbidity and mortality, particularly in hospitals (Aljadhey et al. 2016). Authorities might thus require pharmacists to report adverse events, such as in Saudi Arabia (Aldryhim et al. 2019). In fact, pharmacovigilance systems are being established in the majority of Middle Eastern countries, at different stages of implementation (Alshammari, Mendi, et al. 2019, Wilbur 2013). In some countries like Lebanon, the pharmacovigilance system is not established yet, although pharmacists declared their readiness to participate in adverse events reporting (Hallit, Hajj, Shuhaiber, et al. 2019, Hajj et al. 2018). We also note that underreporting of adverse events is common among Middle Eastern pharmacists, such as in Saudi Arabia due to inadequate knowledge and attitude (Ali et al. 2018); in Syria, the cited reasons for underreporting are uncertainty of the fate of the reports, how they would be addressed, the complexity of the forms and the modest publicity of the pharmacovigilance programme (Bahnassi and Al-Harbi 2018),; similar reasons were also found in Kuwait (Lemay, Alsaleh, et al. 2018).

Underreporting is also common for medication prescribing errors, largely related to emotions and related beliefs of consequences (Stewart, Thomas, MacLure, Wilbur, et al. 2018, Alqubaisi et al. 2016); patient safety inappropriate culture, lack of awareness and insufficiency of reporting by health care professionals, can also be incriminated (Hammoudi, Ismaile, and Abu Yahya 2018), despite the fact irrational prescribing (and thus medication errors) is common in some countries, such as Jordan (Al-Azayzih et al. 2017), Qatar (Pawluk et al. 2017) and Lebanon (Zeenny, Wakim, and Kuyumjian 2017, Sakr et al. 2018). In parallel, medications dispensing errors are inadequately reported and addressed (Shawahna et al. 2016), particularly in hospitals (Salameh et al. 2007).

4.11. Wars, Conflicts, and Political Instability

Wars and conflicts negatively impact all facets of a health system, including pharmacy; services cease to function, resources become depleted and any semblance of governance is lost. Moreover, following cessation of conflict, the rebuilding process includes a wide array of international and local actors that should involve pharmacists (Rutherford and Saleh 2019). On another hand, refugees fleeing these conflicts generally live in precarious conditions that increase morbidity and mortality; pharmacists practicing in affected regions need to be ready for new challenges. Examples include antibiotic resistance issues from Syria spreading to the Middle East (Jakovljevic et al. 2018), high prevalence of antibiotic misuse in refugee camps (Al Baz, Law, and Saadeh 2018), child marriages and contraceptive issues (Bardaweel, Akour, and A 2019). Moreover, refugees may be a burden on medications procurement system; despite the international help received to support health care provision and medications procurement for the refugees, support might not be sufficient and more is needed due to the shortage of some medications (Daher and Alabbadi 2017). Consequently, the intervention of pharmacists in these setting is highly appreciated by both physicians and patients, as it has been reported in Jordan for example (Al Alawneh, Nuaimi, and Basheti 2019). As for Iran, sanctions have had a negative effect on availability and access to drugs, particularly those that depended on the import of their raw material or finished products (Kheirandish et al. 2018).

4.12. Cultural Specificities and Gender Differences

The Middle East still has cultural specificities related mainly to gender, originating in social and religious norms. Arab Muslim women are diverse in their adherence to religious and cultural traditions, with the vast majority adhering based on personal convictions but in some countries based on family pressure and governmental rules (Alsharif et al. 2019). Moreover, the relative frequency of consanguineous marriages in the region, mainly related to cultural and religious customs (Barbour and Salameh 2009), may increase the rates of some diseases considerably, such as neurological, cardiovascular and metabolic diseases (Daher and El-Khairy 2014).

For patients, the Middle East also shows discrepancies in treatment among women as compared to men; this applies to sexual and reproductive health, but also for chronic diseases. For example, diabetic women were less likely to be on optimal hypolipemic therapy and consequently less likely to attain lipid goals compared to men in the Gulf region (Al-Zakwani et al. 2018), although there is a high prevalence of lifestyle-related diseases among women population in the Gulf, considered as a "ticking time bomb" and reaching alarming levels. Therefore, fundamental social and political changes are still required to avoid the deleterious consequences of these diseases on women (Alshaikh et al. 2017). The introduction of "women only" services might be useful in some settings (Alam-mehrjerdi et al. 2016). In Lebanon, elderly women suffer from poor nutritional status, self-perceived health, absence of physical activity, comorbidity, polymedication and depression (as compared to men) (Mitri, Boulos, and Adib 2017).

It is noteworthy to add that the cultural issue also applies to the pharmacist, female graduates facing challenges in the pharmacy workforce, especially in the pharmaceutical sector. Lack of training, job stability, as well as religious and cultural constraints influence female graduate's decision to join a particular sector in the pharmacy field (Al Ghazzawi et al. 2017).

4.13. Environmental Issues Related to Medications Storage and Disposal

Patients commonly store unused medications; however, storage conditions seem inappropriate (Abushanab, Sweileh, and Wazaify 2013). In parallel, many medications' users are unaware about the disposal of unused or expired medicines; gaps exist in practice, due to the lack of robust, safe and cost-effective pharmaceutical waste management program at the national levels and supported with media campaigns. Healthcare practitioners and community pharmacists are not always trained to educate customers on standard disposal practices (Bashaar et al. 2017), and patients have insufficient knowledge about the issue (Al-Shareef et al. 2016). In some countries like Lebanon, there are no safe disposal measures for expired medications; the latter are either returned to the manufacturers or disposed of through domestic sewage pipelines, which exposes the population to chemical pollution and potentially related problems (Massoud et al. 2016).

5. Perspectives and Recommendations

To overcome the abovementioned challenges, several recommendations can be made. Their application is likely to improve pharmacy education, research and practice in the Middle East.

5.1. Governance Principles in the Pharmaceutical Sector

Health system governance elements including strategic vision, participation, transparency, responsiveness, equity, effectiveness, accountability, and information should be applied to the pharmacy sector. As governance application is weak in the institutions of the region, such an application to the pharmaceutical sector was locally suggested by the Lebanese Order of Pharmacists to manage several difficulties the profession in facing in Lebanon (Sacre, Hallit, et al. 2019). The international community must specifically focus on increasing government efficacy and improving accountability, which can both lead to reform that will in turn expand and protect opportunities, decrease mortality and improve health and well-being in the region (Batniji et al. 2014).

5.2. Developing Appropriate Strategic Plans

Although professional pharmacy organizations in the region tend to take on a political nature at education and practice levels (Alsharif et al. 2019, Hallit, Sacre, Hajj, et al. 2019), potential strategies have to be developed for improving the quality of education and expanding pharmacy practice to ensure graduates and practitioners have adequate experiential opportunities and institutional support (Al-Ghananeem et al. 2018, Sacre, Hallit, et al. 2019).

New approaches and frameworks, such as those developed by international authorities in pharmacy (FIP), might be useful: the Nanjing statements stress on investing in workforce development to improve population health and economic well-being, improving health systems access to needed medicines, optimizing medicines use and reducing their associated risk (Baines et al. 2018). International guidelines, along with national and local strategic plans, need to be implemented, as the case of Jordan: new conceptual frameworks of interrelated professional sectors (education, research, regulation and practice) would allow for identification and resolving of challenges facing the pharmacy profession (Bader et al. 2017).

5.3. Adopting Quality Standards for Modern Education

This process would start by the elaboration of core and specific competencies frameworks for different sectors of pharmacy to guide bridging the gap between education and practice (Bajis et al. 2016). Governmental and educational institutions should also recognize and consider specialized competencies and degrees (Hallit S et al. 2018, Hammad, Al Akhali, and Elsobky); these endeavors should be undertaken in the light of quality standards (Bajis et al. 2018). Universities offering pharmacy programs should seek accreditation from national or international bodies to ensure they are within accepted international quality standards (Alhamoudi and Alnattah 2018). The assessment processes currently used to evaluate competencies may need to be enhanced, through the use of well-designed rubrics, standardized scales or other strategies to empower respondents and subsequently improve their ability to self-assess their competencies (Kheir, Al-Ismail, and Al-Nakeeb 2017).

5.4. Applying Interprofessional Education Principles

Effective strategies for the integration and enhancement of IPE to promote collaborative education, collaboration, and communication are important concepts to be applied in appropriate settings. Roles of different health professionals should be clearly established at the national levels. IPE can contribute to improving communication and collaboration between health professions, including the pharmacists, as suggested in some countries (El-Awaisi et al. 2019). The positive perceptions towards IPE suggest a high level of support and an opportunity for pharmacy academics to drive the IPE agenda forward in Qatar and maybe other countries (El-Awaisi et al. 2019). In fact, some success stories have been reported in the region, such as in Lebanon (Farra et al. 2018) and Qatar (El-Awaisi, Wilby, et al. 2017). A positive change in perception was also noted following an IPE activity in Qatar, indicating the effectiveness and the value of even short duration IPE activities in negating usual harmful stereotypical views (El-Awaisi et al. 2020). Furthermore, IPE could be used for any pharmacy or health related topic of interest, such as reported in Qatar for smoking cessation (El-Awaisi, Awaisu, et al. 2017).

5.5. Adopting and Implementing Good Pharmacy Practice Quality Standards

Quality standards developed by international authorities exist for both community and hospital pharmacy, but are still weakly implemented in the Middle Eastern region. An initiative was taken in Lebanon by the Lebanese Order of Pharmacists, but still without implementation (Hallit, Sacre, Sarkis, et al. 2019); related baseline assessment of community pharmacists' readiness to implement the Good Pharmacy Practice standards showed a profound need to homogenize practice in several domains (Badro DA et al. 2020 Mar). Standardized methods can also be used to apply quality standards and clinical guidelines in practice (Babiker et al. 2018). Finally, adaptation of international standards are suggested to facilitate their implementation in local settings, such as the simplification of Basel Statements for hospital pharmacy (Al Sabban et al. 2018).

5.6. Applying Innovative Methods in Manufacturing Products

In addition to internationally adopted good manufacturing practice standards, some additional processes could be used in the region, responding to specific needs. For example, adapting medication labels to low literacy individuals is necessary, whereby simple pictorials supported by verbal instructions were better comprehended by individuals with low literacy skills than labels with written plus verbal instructions in a language that the individual did not understand (Kheir et al. 2014).

5.7. Applying Innovative and Bold Practice Concepts

5.7.1. Medication Reconciliation

Pharmacy-led medication reconciliation upon hospital admission, along with student pharmacist involvement and physician communication can reduce unintended discrepancies and improve medication safety and patient outcomes in a Lebanese hospital (Karaoui et al. 2019). It can also reduce medication related preventable adverse events, as shown in Oman (Al-Hashar et al. 2018) or Saudi Arabia (Abdulghani et al. 2018). Related to medication reconciliation is the practice of de-prescribing, that should be conducted in collaboration with physicians, particularly for elderly (AlRasheed et al. 2018). Policy reforms and teams trainings are however necessary to be able to apply these relatively new and useful practices (Katoue and Ker 2018).

5.7.2. Pharmacists' Prescribing

An accumulation of international evidence demonstrates that pharmacist prescribing is effective, safe and well-accepted, for minor ailments in particular. The need for further training, demonstration of pharmacists' prescribing competence, and extensive engagement of stakeholders were considered crucial for the establishment of this system in Qatar (Jebara et al. 2019). In some cases, the cost effectiveness of over-the-counter drug delivery has been demonstrated (Amirsadri and Hassani 2015).

5.7.3. Improvement of Adverse Events Reporting by Pharmacists

To increase reporting by pharmacists, the most important factors include ongoing improvements in therapeutic knowledge about adverse reactions, attending educational programs with continuous medical education credits, showing the seriousness of the experienced adverse reactions and increasing accessibility to patients' medical profile (Aldryhim et al. 2019). The concept of medication safety should even be educated to pharmacy students well before graduation (Aldossary 2019).

5.7.4. Health Promotion and Disease Prevention Activation

Pharmacists of the region should be ready for activities that promote health and prevent disease, particularly improving vaccines coverage such as flu and other infectious diseases (Al Awaidy et al. 2018). Given that vaccine hesitancy is becoming more common in some Muslim countries, there is a major role for pharmacists in decreasing the incidence of vaccine preventable diseases through patients' advice (Ahmed et al. 2018).

5.7.5. Clinical Pharmacy and Interprofessional Collaboration in Pharmacy Settings

Recommendations concerning a wide variety of drug related problems and different classes of drugs indicate that advanced collaboration among physicians, nurses and pharmacists is possible in interdisciplinary assessment teams. Clinical pharmacy services can thus be instrumental in several settings where advice about medications is needed, such as in a hospital setting (Bayoud et al. 2018), a geriatric ward (Ertuna et al. 2019), a diabetic outpatient setting (Abdulrhim et al. 2019), an internal medicine setting (Haydar et al. 2019), an oncology ward (Bosnak et al. 2019), disease specific clinics (Al-Mahrezi et al. 2018, Elewa, AbdelSamad, et al. 2016, Elewa, Jalali, et al. 2016), or in the community setting (Almomani et al. 2017, Apikoglu-Rabus, Yesilyaprak, and Izzettin 2016).

5.7.6. Medication Therapy Management (MTM)

Given the importance of patient-centered care, pharmacists in the region should be applying Medication Therapy Management (MTM) in the community and in the hospital. In Lebanon for example, Lebanese pharmacists had adequate knowledge and a positive attitude towards medication therapy management services implementation (Domiati et al. 2018). In the Kingdom of Saudi Arabia, residents highly appreciated the additional values of the MTM program if implemented by community pharmacists (Alhaddad 2019). However, in Qatar, many community pharmacists did not show adequate competencies necessary for disease prevention and management services (Zolezzi et al. 2019). Major efforts have to be developed to implement MTM in the region.

5.8. Capacity Building and Continuous Professional Development (CPD)

In fact, capacity building can play an essential role in addressing the major health challenges and improving the overall quality of health care in the region. Efforts aimed at increasing the number of appropriately and locally-trained graduates and developing and implementing need-based CPD programs are vital for capacity building and lifelong learning in health care professions, particularly pharmacy (Sheikh et al. 2019). One major point in continuous professional development of pharmacists is computer literacy, this competency being essential in modern pharmacy and health technology application (Al-Aqeel 2018). Another interesting activity would be to use simulated patients to improve community pharmacists counseling practices, as reported in Qatar (Paravattil, Kheir, and Yousif 2017).

5.9. Setting Research Strategies for Health and Pharmacy in the Region

Although priorities were established in some countries such as Iran (Mansoori et al. 2018), clear research strategies remain to be integrated for the region, to fill out the gaps in knowledge about the region. The strengths, weaknesses, opportunities and challenges of research in the region are to be collaboratively thought of, to come up with a pharmaceutical research strategy that addresses the pharmacy researchers' concerns and promotes patients' health. Pharmacists' professional associations, in collaboration with academia, industry, political authorities and other involved stakeholders, are required to promote research at the local and regional levels (Hallit, Sacre, and Salameh 2019). Policy-makers are encouraged to (i) support the researchers and institutions that have proved research capacity; (ii) direct further resources towards research areas and/or institutions that are lagging behind; (iii) facilitate further international collaboration with the academics and/or institutions that have shown the capacity for conducting successful research projects (Mansoori 2018).

One major gap is in making the case of pharmaceutical services' economic impact, starting by clinical pharmacy services in hospitals to medication therapy management in the community in the region (Eljilany et al. 2018). Another gap is the assessment of effectiveness of medications in Middle Eastern populations, that may differ from western populations due to pharmacogenetic and/or environmental discrepancies (Albassam et al. 2018, Dagenais et al. 2017). Interventional studies are also of utmost importance: for example, although knowledge and attitudes are important contributing factors in the misuse of medications, strategies and interventions to limit misuse were rarely identified in literature. Standardization of studies is a prerequisite to the understanding and prevention of misuse of self-medication (Khalifeh, Moore, and Salameh 2017).

5.10. Assessing the Pharmaceutical System Structure and Processes

The system structure and processes need to be regularly assessed, to evaluate goals' achievement for the pharmacists and the patients, in addition to other health care professionals and institutions (Alefan, Amairi, and Tawalbeh 2018). Suggesting new assessment tools (Yaghoubifard et al. 2015), new approaches and business models might help resolving certain financial and administrative issues: for example, a proposed pricing system based on willingness to pay will help pharmaceutical authorities make realistic price estimates of pharmaceutical products, while accounting for patient preferences, which may enhance patients' adherence to treatment (Rahimi et al. 2018). The use of Managed Entry Agreement is useful in this regard, although not always used due lack of data infrastructure as well as a shortage of experts in health economics (Maskineh and Nasser 2018). Other quality improvement suggestions can also be adopted, according to the national system already in place: partnership between the public and private sectors under government supervision, could represent an acceptable option for addressing the variation in public preferences (Al-Hanawi et al. 2018), increasing transparency and decreasing corruption (Badawi et al. 2015).

CONCLUSION

In conclusion, challenges are numerous and tremendous efforts are required for the improvement of pharmacy in the Middle East; difficulties arise at all levels from education, research to practice. Collaborative assessment of barriers and facilitators, strengths and weaknesses, opportunities and threats, are necessary for strategic planning, adapted to local and regional settings. Potential stakeholders to work on this endeavor are academia (teachers and researchers), professional associations, industrials and health authorities.

REFERENCES

Abdel-Latif, M. M. M., and S. Y. Saad. 2019. "Health literacy among Saudi population: a cross-sectional study." *Health Promot Int* 34 (1):60-70. doi: 10.1093/heapro/dax043.

Abduelkarem, A. R., and H. Mustafa. 2017. "Use of Over-the-Counter Medication among Pregnant Women in Sharjah, United Arab Emirates." *J Pregnancy* 2017:4503793. doi: 10.1155/2017/4503793.

Abdulameer, S. A. 2018. "Knowledge and pharmaceutical care practice regarding inhaled therapy among registered and unregistered pharmacists: an urgent need for a patient-oriented health care educational program in Iraq." *Int J Chron Obstruct Pulmon Dis* 13:879-888. doi: 10.2147/COPD.S157403.

Abdulghani, K. H., M. A. Aseeri, A. Mahmoud, and R. Abulezz. 2018. "The impact of pharmacist-led medication reconciliation during admission at tertiary care hospital." *Int J Clin Pharm* 40 (1):196-201. doi: 10.1007/s11096-017-0568-6.

Abdulrhim, S. H., R. A. Saleh, M. A. Mohamed Hussain, H. Al Raey, A. H. Babiker, N. Kheir, and A. Awaisu. 2019. "Impact of a Collaborative Pharmaceutical Care Service Among Patients With Diabetes in an Ambulatory Care Setting in Qatar: A Multiple Time Series Study." *Value Health Reg Issues* 19:45-50. doi: 10.1016/j.vhri.2018.12.002.

Abood, E. A., and M. Wazaify. 2016. "Abuse and Misuse of Prescription and Nonprescription Drugs from Community Pharmacies in Aden City-Yemen." *Subst Use Misuse* 51 (7):942-7. doi: 10.3109/10826084.2016.1155619.

Abu Farha, R., K. Abu Hammour, S. Al-Jamei, R. AlQudah, and M. Zawiah. 2018. "The prevalence and clinical seriousness of medication discrepancies identified upon hospital admission of pediatric patients." *BMC Health Serv Res* 18 (1):966. doi: 10.1186/s12913-018-3795-1.

Abu Farha, R., E. Alefishat, M. Suyagh, E. Elayeh, and A. Mayyas. 2014. "Evidence-based medicine use in pharmacy practice: a cross-sectional survey." *J Eval Clin Pract* 20 (6):786-92. doi: 10.1111/jep.12212.

Abushanab, A. S., W. M. Sweileh, and M. Wazaify. 2013. "Storage and wastage of drug products in Jordanian households: a cross-sectional survey." *Int J Pharm Pract* 21 (3):185-91. doi: 10.1111/j.2042-7174.2012.00250.x.

Ahmed, A., K. S. Lee, A. Bukhsh, Y. M. Al-Worafi, M. M. R. Sarker, L. C. Ming, and T. M. Khan. 2018. "Outbreak of vaccine-preventable diseases in Muslim majority countries." *J Infect Public Health* 11 (2):153-155. doi: 10.1016/j.jiph.2017.09.007.

Al-Aqeel, S. 2018. "Health technology assessment in Saudi Arabia." *Expert Rev Pharmacoecon Outcomes Res* 18 (4):393-402. doi: 10.1080/14737167.2018.1474102.

Al-Azayzih, A., S. I. Al-Azzam, K. H. Alzoubi, M. Shawaqfeh, and M. M. Masadeh. 2017. "Evaluation of drug-prescribing patterns based on the WHO prescribing indicators at outpatient clinics of five hospitals in Jordan: a cross-sectional study." *Int J Clin Pharmacol Ther* 55 (5):425-432. doi: 10.5414/CP202733.

Al-Ghananeem, A. M., D. R. Malcom, S. Shammas, and T. Aburjai. 2018. "A Call to Action to Transform Pharmacy Education and Practice in the Arab World." *Am J Pharm Educ* 82 (9):7014. doi: 10.5688/ajpe 7014.

Al-Hanawi, M. K., O. Alsharqi, S. Almazrou, and K. Vaidya. 2018. "Healthcare Finance in the Kingdom of Saudi Arabia: A Qualitative Study of Householders' Attitudes." *Appl Health Econ Health Policy* 16 (1):55-64. doi: 10.1007/s40258-017-0353-7.

Al-Hashar, A., I. Al-Zakwani, T. Eriksson, A. Sarakbi, B. Al-Zadjali, S. Al Mubaihsi, and M. Al Za'abi. 2018. "Impact of medication reconciliation and review and counselling, on adverse drug events and healthcare resource use." *Int J Clin Pharm* 40 (5):1154-1164. doi: 10.1007/s11096-018-0650-8.

Al-Jumaili, A. A., M. D. Al-Rekabi, O. S. Alsawad, O. Q. B. Allela, R. Carnahan, H. Saaed, A. Naqishbandi, D. J. Kadhim, and B. Sorofman. 2017. "Exploring Electronic Communication Modes Between Iraqi Faculty and Students of Pharmacy Schools Using the Technology Acceptance Model." *Am J Pharm Educ* 81 (5):89. doi: 10.5688/ajpe 81589.

Al-Jumaili, A. A., M. D. Al-Rekabi, W. Doucette, A. H. Hussein, H. K. Abbas, and F. H. Hussein. 2017. "Factors influencing the degree of physician-pharmacist collaboration within Iraqi public healthcare settings." *Int J Pharm Pract* 25 (6):411-417. doi: 10.1111/ijpp.12339.

Al-Mahrezi, A., S. Baddar, S. Al-Siyabi, S. Al-Kindi, I. Al-Zakwani, and O. Al-Rawas. 2018. "Asthma Clinics in Primary Healthcare Centres in Oman: Do they make a difference?" *Sultan Qaboos Univ Med J* 18 (2):e137-e142. doi: 10.18295/squmj.2018.18.02.003.

Al-Qadheeb, N. S., D. A. Alissa, A. Al-Jedai, A. Ajlan, and A. S. Al-Jazairi. 2012. "The first international residency program accredited by the American Society of Health-System Pharmacists." *Am J Pharm Educ* 76 (10):190. doi: 10.5688/ajpe7610190.

Al-Shareef, F., S. A. El-Asrar, L. Al-Bakr, M. Al-Amro, F. Alqahtani, F. Aleanizy, and S. Al-Rashood. 2016. "Investigating the disposal of expired and unused medication in Riyadh, Saudi Arabia: a cross-sectional study." *Int J Clin Pharm* 38 (4):822-8. doi: 10.1007/s11096-016-0287-4.

Al-Tamimi, S. K., M. A. Hassali, A. A. Shafie, and A. Lrasheedy AA. 2016. "The need to incorporate generic medicines topic in the curriculum of Yemeni pharmacy colleges." *Int J Pharm Pract* 24 (1):72-3. doi: 10.1111/ijpp.12204.

Al-Worafi, Yaser Mohammed, Rahul P Patel, Syed Tabish Razi Zaidi, Wafa Mohammed Alseragi, Masaad Saeed Almutairi, Ali Saleh Alkhoshaiban, and Long Chiau Ming. 2018. "Completeness and legibility of handwritten prescriptions in Sana'a, Yemen." *Medical Principles and Practice* 27:290-292.

Al-Zakwani, I., F. Al-Mahruqi, K. Al-Rasadi, A. Shehab, W. Al Mahmeed, M. Arafah, A. T. Al-Hinai, O. Al Tamimi, M. Al Awadhi, and R. D. Santos. 2018. "Sex disparity in the management and outcomes of dyslipidemia of diabetic patients in the Arabian Gulf: findings from the CEPHEUS study." *Lipids Health Dis* 17 (1):25. doi: 10.1186/s12944-018-0667-y.

Al Alawneh, M., N. Nuaimi, and I. A. Basheti. 2019. "Pharmacists in humanitarian crisis settings: Assessing the impact of pharmacist-delivered home medication management review service to Syrian refugees in Jordan." *Res Social Adm Pharm* 15 (2):164-172. doi: 10.1016/j.sapharm.2018.04.008.

Al Awaidy, S., A. Althaqafi, G. Dbaibo, and Network Middle East/North Africa Influenza Stakeholder. 2018. "A Snapshot of Influenza Surveillance, Vaccine Recommendations, and Vaccine Access, Drivers, and Barriers in Selected Middle Eastern and North African Countries." *Oman Med J* 33 (4):283-290. doi: 10.5001/omj.2018.54.

Al Baz, M., M. R. Law, and R. Saadeh. 2018. "Antibiotics use among Palestine refugees attending UNRWA primary health care centers in Jordan - A cross-sectional study." *Travel Med Infect Dis* 22:25-29. doi: 10.1016/j.tmaid.2018.02.004.

Al Ghazzawi, W. F., A. Abuzaid, O. A. Al-Shareef, and S. M. Al-Sayagh. 2017. "Female pharmacists' career perceptions in Saudi Arabia: A survey at an academic center in Jeddah." *Curr Pharm Teach Learn* 9 (6):1022-1030. doi: 10.1016/j.cptl.2017.07.010.

Al Juffali, L., S. Al-Aqeel, P. Knapp, K. Mearns, H. Family, and M. Watson. 2019. "Using the Human Factors Framework to understand the origins of medication safety problems in community pharmacy: A qualitative study." *Res Social Adm Pharm* 15 (5):558-567. doi: 10.1016/j.sapharm.2018.07.010.

Al Khalidi, D., and M. Wazaify. 2013. "Assessment of pharmacists' job satisfaction and job related stress in Amman." *Int J Clin Pharm* 35 (5):821-8. doi: 10.1007/s11096-013-9815-7.

Al Sabban, H., A. Al-Jedai, D. Bajis, and J. Penm. 2018. "The Revised Basel Statements on the Future of Hospital Pharmacy: What Do They Mean for Saudi Arabia?" *Int J Pharm Pract* 26 (3):281-283. doi: 10.1111/ijpp.12394.

Alam-mehrjerdi, Z., R. Daneshmand, M. Samiei, R. Samadi, M. Abdollahi, and K. Dolan. 2016. "Women-only drug treatment services and needs in Iran: the first review of current literature." *Daru* 24:3. doi: 10.1186/s40199-016-0141-1.

Alaqeel, S., and N. O. Abanmy. 2015. "Counselling practices in community pharmacies in Riyadh, Saudi Arabia: a cross-sectional study." *BMC Health Serv Res* 15:557. doi: 10.1186/s12913-015-1220-6.

Albassam, A., S. Alshammari, G. Ouda, S. Koshy, and A. Awad. 2018. "Knowledge, perceptions and confidence of physicians and pharmacists towards pharmacogenetics practice in Kuwait." *PLoS One* 13 (9):e0203033. doi: 10.1371/journal.pone.0203033.

Albassam, A., and A. Awad. 2018. "Community pharmacists' services for women during pregnancy and breast feeding in Kuwait: a cross-sectional study." *BMJ Open* 8 (1):e018980. doi: 10.1136/bmjopen-2017-018980.

Alburikan, K. A., A. AbuAlreesh, M. Alenazi, H. Albabtain, M. Alqouzi, M. Alawaji, and H. S. Aljadhey. 2018. "Patients' understanding of prescription drug label instructions in developing nations: The case of Saudi Arabia." *Res Social Adm Pharm* 14 (5):413-417. doi: 10.1016/j.sapharm.2017.05.004.

Aldohyan, M., N. Al-Rawashdeh, F. M. Sakr, S. Rahman, A. I. Alfarhan, and M. Salam. 2019. "The perceived effectiveness of MERS-CoV educational programs and knowledge transfer among primary healthcare workers: a cross-sectional survey." *BMC Infect Dis* 19 (1):273. doi: 10.1186/s12879-019-3898-2.

Aldossary, S. A. 2019. "Patient safety attitudes of clinical Pharmacy Students attending undergraduate program in King Faisal University." *Pak J Pharm Sci* 32 (1(Special)):471-475.

Aldryhim, A. Y., A. Alomair, M. Alqhtani, M. A. Mahmoud, T. M. Alshammari, L. G. Pont, K. M. Kamal, H. Aljadhey, A. B. Mekonnen, M. Alwhaibi, B. Balkhi, and T. M. Alhawassi. 2019. "Factors that facilitate reporting of adverse drug reactions by pharmacists in Saudi Arabia." *Expert Opin Drug Saf* 18 (8):745-752. doi: 10.1080/14740338.2019.1632287.

Alefan, Q., R. Amairi, and S. Tawalbeh. 2018. "Availability, prices and affordability of selected essential medicines in Jordan: a national survey." *BMC Health Serv Res* 18 (1):787. doi: 10.1186/s12913-018-3593-9.

Alghamdi, S., N. A. Shebl, Z. Aslanpour, A. Shibl, and I. Berrou. 2018. "Hospital adoption of antimicrobial stewardship programmes in Gulf Cooperation Council countries: A review of existing evidence." *J Glob Antimicrob Resist* 15:196-209. doi: 10.1016/j.jgar.2018.07.014.

Alhaddad, M. S., Q. M. Abdallah, S. M. Alshakhsheer, S. B. Alosaimi, A. R. Althmali, and S. A. Alahmari. 2014. "General public knowledge, preferred dosage forms, and beliefs toward medicines in western Saudi Arabia." *Saudi Med J* 35 (6):578-84.

Alhaddad, Mahmoud S. 2019. "Youth Experience With Community Pharmacy Services and Their Perceptions Toward Implementation of Medication Therapy Management Services by Community Pharmacists in the Western Region of Saudi Arabia." *Therapeutic innovation & regulatory science* 53 (1):95-99.

Alhamoudi, A., and A. Alnattah. 2018. "Pharmacy education in Saudi Arabia: The past, the present, and the future." *Curr Pharm Teach Learn* 10 (1):54-60. doi: 10.1016/j.cptl.2017.09.014.

Alhomoud, F., Z. Aljamea, R. Almahasnah, K. Alkhalifah, L. Basalelah, and F. K. Alhomoud. 2017. "Self-medication and self-prescription with antibiotics in the Middle East-do they really happen? A systematic review of the prevalence, possible reasons, and outcomes." *Int J Infect Dis* 57:3-12. doi: 10.1016/j.ijid.2017.01.014.

Alhomoud, F., Z. Aljamea, and L. Basalelah. 2018. ""Antibiotics kill things very quickly" - consumers' perspectives on non-prescribed antibiotic use in Saudi Arabia." *BMC Public Health* 18 (1):1177. doi: 10.1186/s12889-018-6088-z.

Alhomoud, F., R. Almahasnah, and F. K. Alhomoud. 2018. ""You could lose when you misuse" - factors affecting over-the-counter sale of antibiotics in community pharmacies in Saudi Arabia: a qualitative study." *BMC Health Serv Res* 18 (1):915. doi: 10.1186/s12913-018-3753-y.

Ali, M. D., Y. A. Hassan, A. Ahmad, O. Alaqel, H. Al-Harbi, and N. M. Al-Suhaimi. 2018. "Knowledge, Practice and Attitudes Toward Pharmacovigilance and Adverse Drug Reactions Reporting Process Among Health Care Providers in Dammam, Saudi Arabia." *Curr Drug Saf* 13 (1):21-25. doi: 10.2174/1574886313666171218123802.

Alipour, F., F. Peiravian, and G. Mehralian. 2018. "Perceptions, experiences and expectations of physicians regarding the role of pharmacists in low-income and middle-income countries: the case of Tehran hospital settings." *BMJ Open* 8 (2):e019237. doi: 10.1136/bmjopen-2017-019237.

Aljadani, R., and M. Aseeri. 2018. "Prevalence of drug-drug interactions in geriatric patients at an ambulatory care pharmacy in a tertiary care teaching hospital." *BMC Res Notes* 11 (1):234. doi: 10.1186/s13104-018-3342-5.

Aljadhey, H., M. A. Mahmoud, Y. Ahmed, R. Sultana, S. Zouein, S. Alshanawani, A. Mayet, M. K. Alshaikh, N. Kalagi, E. Al Tawil, A. R. El Kinge, A. Arwadi, M. Alyahya, M. D. Murray, and D. Bates. 2016. "Incidence of adverse drug events in public and private hospitals in Riyadh, Saudi Arabia: the (ADESA) prospective cohort study." *BMJ Open* 6 (7):e010831. doi: 10.1136/bmjopen-2015-010831.

Alkhateeb, F. M., S. Arkle, S. L. K. McDonough, and D. A. Latif. 2018. "Review of National and International Accreditation of Pharmacy Programs in the Gulf Cooperation Council Countries." *Am J Pharm Educ* 82 (10):5980. doi: 10.5688/ajpe5980.

Alkhuzaee, F. S., H. M. Almalki, A. Y. Attar, S. I. Althubiani, W. A. Almuallim, E. Cheema, and M. A. Hadi. 2016. "Evaluating community pharmacists' perspectives and practices concerning generic medicines substitution in Saudi Arabia: A cross-sectional study." *Health Policy* 120 (12):1412-1419. doi: 10.1016/j.healthpol.2016.09.018.

Alluqmani, W. S., M. M. Alotaibi, W. J. Almalki, A. Althaqafi, H. A. Alawi, F. Althobiani, A. A. Albishi, A. A. Madkhali, L. Y. Baunes, R. I. Alhazmi, E. M. Doman, A. H. Alhazmi, M. Ali, and E. Cheema. 2019. "Exploring Drug-Related Problems in Diabetic Patients during Ramadan Fasting in Saudi Arabia: A Mixed-Methods Study." *Int J Environ Res Public Health* 16 (3). doi: 10.3390/ijerph16030499.

Almaghaslah, D., A. Alsayari, R. Asiri, and N. Albugami. 2019. "Pharmacy workforce in Saudi Arabia: Challenges and opportunities: A cross-sectional study." *Int J Health Plann Manage* 34 (1):e583-e593. doi: 10.1002/hpm.2674.

Almalag, H. M., H. Alzahrani, F. Al-Hussain, A. Alsemari, E. B. De Vol, M. R. Almarzouqi, and Y. S. AlRuthia. 2018. "The impact of old versus new antiepileptic drugs on costs and patient reported outcomes among older adults." *Geriatr Nurs* 39 (6):669-675. doi: 10.1016/j.gerinurse.2018.05.001.

Almomani, B. A., R. K. Mayyas, F. A. Ekteish, A. M. Ayoub, M. A. Ababneh, and S. A. Alzoubi. 2017. "The effectiveness of clinical pharmacist's intervention in improving asthma care in children and adolescents: Randomized controlled study in Jordan." *Patient Educ Couns* 100 (4):728-735. doi: 10.1016/j.pec.2016.11.002.

Alqubaisi, M., A. Tonna, A. Strath, and D. Stewart. 2016. "Exploring behavioural determinants relating to health professional reporting of medication errors: a qualitative study using the Theoretical Domains Framework." *Eur J Clin Pharmacol* 72 (7):887-95. doi: 10.1007/s00228-016-2054-9.

AlRasheed, M. M., T. M. Alhawassi, A. Alanazi, N. Aloudah, F. Khurshid, and M. Alsultan. 2018. "Knowledge and willingness of physicians about deprescribing among older patients: a qualitative study." *Clin Interv Aging* 13:1401-1408. doi: 10.2147/CIA.S165588.

Alrasheedy, A. A., M. A. Hassali, H. Aljadhey, and S. K. Al-Tamimi. 2014. "The need to cover generic medications and generic substitution practice in the curricula of pharmacy colleges in Saudi Arabia." *Am J Pharm Educ* 78 (5):108. doi: 10.5688/ajpe785108.

AlRuthia, Y., S. Alhawas, F. Alodaibi, L. Almutairi, R. Algasem, H. K. Alrabiah, I. Sales, H. Alsobayel, and Y. Ghawaa. 2019. "The use of active learning strategies in healthcare colleges in the Middle East." *BMC Med Educ* 19 (1):143. doi: 10.1186/s12909-019-1580-4.

Alsaleh, F. M., E. A. Abahussain, H. H. Altabaa, M. F. Al-Bazzaz, and N. B. Almandil. 2018. "Assessment of patient safety culture: a nationwide survey of community pharmacists in Kuwait." *BMC Health Serv Res* 18 (1):884. doi: 10.1186/s12913-018-3662-0.

Alshaikh, M. K., F. T. Filippidis, H. A. Al-Omar, S. Rawaf, A. Majeed, and A. M. Salmasi. 2017. "The ticking time bomb in lifestyle-related diseases among women in the Gulf Cooperation Council countries; review of systematic reviews." *BMC Public Health* 17 (1):536. doi: 10.1186/s12889-017-4331-7.

Alshammari, T. M., N. Mendi, K. A. Alenzi, and Y. Alsowaida. 2019. "Pharmacovigilance Systems in Arab Countries: Overview of 22 Arab Countries." *Drug Saf* 42 (7):849-868. doi: 10.1007/s40264-019-00807-4.

Alshammari, T. M., K. B. Yusuff, M. M. Aziz, and G. M. Subaie. 2019. "Healthcare professionals' knowledge, attitude and acceptance of influenza vaccination in Saudi Arabia: a multicenter cross-sectional study." *BMC Health Serv Res* 19 (1):229. doi: 10.1186/s12913-019-4054-9.

Alsharif, N. Z., N. M. Khanfar, L. F. Brennan, E. B. Chahine, A. M. Al-Ghananeem, J. Retallick, M. Schaalan, and N. Sarhan. 2019. "Cultural Sensitivity and Global Pharmacy Engagement in the Arab World." *Am J Pharm Educ* 83 (4):7228. doi: 10.5688/ajpe7228.

Alsous, M., F. Alhalaiqa, R. Abu Farha, M. Abdel Jalil, J. McElnay, and R. Horne. 2017. "Reliability and validity of Arabic translation of Medication Adherence Report Scale (MARS) and Beliefs about Medication Questionnaire (BMQ)-specific for use in children and their parents." *PLoS One* 12 (2):e0171863. doi: 10.1371/journal.pone.0171863.

Alzubaidi, H., W. Saidawi, and K. Mc Namara. 2018. "Pharmacist views and pharmacy capacity to deliver professional services in the United Arab Emirates." *Int J Clin Pharm* 40 (5):1106-1115. doi: 10.1007/s11096-018-0662-4.

Amirsadri, M., and A. Hassani. 2015. "Cost-effectiveness and cost-utility analysis of OTC use of simvastatin 10 mg for the primary prevention of myocardial infarction in Iranian men." *Daru* 23:56. doi: 10.1186/s40199-015-0129-2.

Apikoglu-Rabus, S., G. Yesilyaprak, and F. V. Izzettin. 2016. "Drug-related problems and pharmacist interventions in a cohort of patients with asthma and chronic obstructive pulmonary disease." *Respir Med* 120:109-115. doi: 10.1016/j.rmed.2016.10.006.

Assali, M., A. Shakaa, S. Abu-Hejleh, R. Abu-Omar, N. Karajeh, N. Ajory, S. Zyoud, and W. Sweileh. 2018. "A cross-sectional study of the availability and pharmacist's knowledge of nano-pharmaceutical drugs in Palestinian hospitals." *BMC Health Serv Res* 18 (1):250. doi: 10.1186/s12913-018-3060-7.

Awad, A., A. Al-Haqan, and P. Moreau. 2017. "Motivations, career aspiration, and learning experience of students in the pharmacy program at Kuwait University: A tool to guide curriculum development." *Curr Pharm Teach Learn* 9 (2):332-338. doi: 10.1016/j.cptl.2016.11.018.

Awad, A. I., A. Al-Rasheedi, and J. Lemay. 2017. "Public Perceptions, Expectations, and Views of Community Pharmacy Practice in Kuwait." *Med Princ Pract* 26 (5):438-446. doi: 10.1159/000481662.

Ayoub, S. W., A. H. Musalam, and A. A. Abu Mahadi. 2017. "Drug utilization in primary healthcare centres in the Gaza Strip." *East Mediterr Health J* 23 (10):649-656. doi: 10.26719/2017.23.10.649.

Babiker, A., Y. S. Amer, M. E. Osman, A. Al-Eyadhy, S. Fatani, S. Mohamed, A. Alnemri, M. A. Titi, F. Shaikh, K. A. Alswat, H. A. Wahabi, and L. A. Al-Ansary. 2018. "Failure Mode and Effect Analysis (FMEA) may enhance implementation of clinical practice guidelines: An experience from the Middle East." *J Eval Clin Pract* 24 (1):206-211. doi: 10.1111/jep.12873.

Babiker, A. H., L. Carson, and A. Awaisu. 2014. "Medication use review in Qatar: are community pharmacists prepared for the extended professional role?" *Int J Clin Pharm* 36 (6):1241-50. doi: 10.1007/s11096-014-0025-8.

Badawi, D. A., Y. Alkhamis, M. Qaddoumi, and K. Behbehani. 2015. "National transparency assessment of Kuwait's pharmaceutical sector." *Health Policy* 119 (9):1275-83. doi: 10.1016/j.healthpol.2015.07.001.

Bader, L. R., S. McGrath, M. J. Rouse, and C. Anderson. 2017. "A conceptual framework toward identifying and analyzing challenges to the advancement of pharmacy." *Res Social Adm Pharm* 13 (2):321-331. doi: 10.1016/j.sapharm.2016.03.001.

Badro DA, Sacre H, Hallit S, Amhaz A, and Salameh P. 2020 Mar. "Good pharmacy practice assessment among community pharmacies in Lebanon." *Pharmacy Practice* 16;18 (1):1745.

Bahnassi, A., and F. Al-Harbi. 2018. "Syrian pharmacovigilance system: a survey of pharmacists' knowledge, attitudes and practices." *East Mediterr Health J* 24 (6):569-578. doi: 10.26719/2018.24.6.569.

Baines, D., I. Bates, L. Bader, C. Hale, and P. Schneider. 2018. "Conceptualising production, productivity and technology in pharmacy practice: a novel framework for policy, education and research." *Hum Resour Health* 16 (1):51. doi: 10.1186/s12960-018-0317-5.

Bajis, D., B. Chaar, J. Penm, and R. Moles. 2016. "Competency-based pharmacy education in the Eastern Mediterranean Region-A scoping review." *Curr Pharm Teach Learn* 8 (3):401-428. doi: 10.1016/j.cptl.2016.02.003.

Bajis, D., R. Moles, D. Hosp, and B. Chaar. 2018. "Stakeholders' Perspectives on Quality Assurance of Pharmacy Education in the Eastern Mediterranean Region." *Am J Pharm Educ* 82 (10):6482. doi: 10.5688/ajpe6482.

Barbour, B., and P. Salameh. 2009. "Consanguinity in Lebanon: prevalence, distribution and determinants." *J Biosoc Sci* 41 (4):505-17. doi: 10.1017/S0021932009003290.

Bardaweel, S. K., A. A. Akour, and A. Lkhawaldeh A. 2019. "Impediments to use of oral contraceptives among refugee women in camps, Jordan." *Women Health* 59 (3):252-265. doi: 10.1080/03630242.2018.1452837.

Bashaar, M., V. Thawani, M. A. Hassali, and F. Saleem. 2017. "Disposal practices of unused and expired pharmaceuticals among general public in Kabul." *BMC Public Health* 17 (1):45. doi: 10.1186/s12889-016-3975-z.

Bates, I., C. John, P. Seegobin, and A. Bruno. 2018. "An analysis of the global pharmacy workforce capacity trends from 2006 to 2012." *Hum Resour Health* 16 (1):3. doi: 10.1186/s12960-018-0267-y.

Batniji, R., L. Khatib, M. Cammett, J. Sweet, S. Basu, A. Jamal, P. Wise, and R. Giacaman. 2014. "Governance and health in the Arab world." *Lancet* 383 (9914):343-55. doi: 10.1016/S0140-6736(13)62185-6.

Bayoud, T., M. Waheedi, J. Lemay, and A. Awad. 2018. "Drug therapy problems identification by clinical pharmacists in a private hospital in Kuwait." *Ann Pharm Fr* 76 (3):210-217. doi: 10.1016/j.pharma.2018.01.002.

Bello, A. K., M. Alrukhaimi, G. E. Ashuntantang, E. Bellorin-Font, M. Benghanem Gharbi, B. Braam, J. Feehally, D. C. Harris, V. Jha, K. Jindal, D. W. Johnson, K. Kalantar-Zadeh, R. Kazancioglu, P. G. Kerr, M. Lunney, T. O. Olanrewaju, M. A. Osman, J. Perl, H. U. Rashid, A. Rateb, E. Rondeau, A. M. Sakajiki, A. Samimi, L. Sola, I. Tchokhonelidze, N. Wiebe, C. W. Yang, F. Ye, A. Zemchenkov, M. H. Zhao, and A. Levin. 2018. "Global overview of health systems oversight and financing for kidney care." *Kidney Int Suppl (2011)* 8 (2):41-51. doi: 10.1016/j.kisu.2017.10.008.

Bosnak, A. S., N. Birand, O. Diker, A. Abdi, and B. Basgut. 2019. "The role of the pharmacist in the multidisciplinary approach to the prevention and resolution of drug-related problems in cancer chemotherapy." *J Oncol Pharm Pract* 25 (6):1312-1320. doi: 10.1177/1078155218786048.

Buabbas, A. J., F. M. Alsaleh, H. M. Al-Shawaf, A. Abdullah, and A. Almajran. 2018. "The readiness of hospital pharmacists in Kuwait to practise evidence-based medicine: a cross-sectional study." *BMC Med Inform Decis Mak* 18 (1):4. doi: 10.1186/s12911-018-0585-y.

Dagenais, R., K. J. Wilby, H. Elewa, and M. H. H. Ensom. 2017. "Impact of Genetic Polymorphisms on Phenytoin Pharmacokinetics and Clinical Outcomes in the Middle East and North Africa Region." *Drugs R D* 17 (3):341-361. doi: 10.1007/s40268-017-0195-7.

Daher, A., and I. Alabbadi. 2017. "Investigating the Effect of Syrian Refugees on the Pharmaceutical Sector in Jordan." *Arch Iran Med* 20 (8):538-546.

Daher, S., and L. El-Khairy. 2014. "Association of cerebral palsy with consanguineous parents and other risk factors in a Palestinian population." *East Mediterr Health J* 20 (7):459-68.

Domiati, S., H. Sacre, N. Lahoud, G. Sili, and P. Salameh. 2018. "Knowledge of and readiness for medication therapy management among community pharmacists in Lebanon." *Int J Clin Pharm* 40 (5):1165-1174. doi: 10.1007/s11096-018-0666-0.

El-Awaisi, A., A. Awaisu, M. S. El Hajj, B. Alemrayat, G. Al-Jayyousi, N. Wong, and M. A. Verjee. 2017. "Delivering Tobacco Cessation Content in the Middle East Through Interprofessional Learning." *Am J Pharm Educ* 81 (5):91. doi: 10.5688/ajpe81591.

El-Awaisi, A., A. Awaisu, M. Jaam, M. Saffouh El Hajj, and M. A. Verjee. 2020. "Does the delivery of interprofessional education have an effect on stereotypical views of healthcare students in Qatar?" *J Interprof Care* 34 (1):44-49. doi: 10.1080/13561820.2019.1612863.

El-Awaisi, A., M. S. El Hajj, S. Joseph, and L. Diack. 2018. "Perspectives of practising pharmacists towards interprofessional education and collaborative practice in Qatar." *Int J Clin Pharm* 40 (5):1388-1401. doi: 10.1007/s11096-018-0686-9.

El-Awaisi, A., S. Joseph, M. S. El Hajj, and L. Diack. 2019. "Pharmacy academics' perspectives toward interprofessional Education prior to its implementation in Qatar: a qualitative study." *BMC Med Educ* 19 (1):278. doi: 10.1186/s12909-019-1689-5.

El-Awaisi, A., M. Saffouh El Hajj, S. Joseph, and L. Diack. 2016. "Interprofessional education in the Arabic-speaking Middle East: Perspectives of pharmacy academics." *J Interprof Care* 30 (6):769-776. doi: 10.1080/13561820.2016.1218830.

El-Awaisi, A., K. J. Wilby, K. Wilbur, M. S. El Hajj, A. Awaisu, and B. Paravattil. 2017. "A Middle Eastern journey of integrating Interprofessional Education into the healthcare curriculum: a SWOC analysis." *BMC Med Educ* 17 (1):15. doi: 10.1186/s12909-016-0852-5.

El-Jardali, F., R. Fadlallah, R. Z. Morsi, N. Hemadi, M. Al-Gibbawi, M. Haj, S. Khalil, Y. Saklawi, D. Jamal, and E. A. Akl. 2017. "Pharmacists' views and reported practices in relation to a new generic drug substitution policy in Lebanon: a mixed methods study." *Implement Sci* 12 (1):23. doi: 10.1186/s13012-017-0556-1.

El-Mowafi, I. M., and A. M. Foster. 2019. "Emergency contraception in Jordan: Assessing retail pharmacists' awareness, opinions, and perceptions of need." *Contraception*. doi: 10.1016/j.contraception. 2019.10.002.

El Hajj, M. S., A. Awaisu, N. Kheir, M. H. N. Mohamed, R. S. Haddad, R. A. Saleh, N. M. Alhamad, A. M. Almulla, and Z. R. Mahfoud. 2019. "Evaluation of an intensive education program on the treatment of tobacco-use disorder for pharmacists: a study protocol for a randomized controlled trial." *Trials* 20 (1):25. doi: 10.1186/s13063-018-3068-7.

Elewa, H., D. Alkhiyami, D. Alsahan, and A. Abdel-Aziz. 2015. "A survey on the awareness and attitude of pharmacists and doctors towards the application of pharmacogenomics and its challenges in Qatar." *J Eval Clin Pract* 21 (4):703-9. doi: 10.1111/jep.12372.

Elewa, H. F., O. AbdelSamad, A. E. Elmubark, H. M. Al-Taweel, A. Mohamed, N. Kheir, M. I. Mohamed Ibrahim, and A. Awaisu. 2016. "The first pharmacist-managed anticoagulation clinic under a collaborative practice agreement in Qatar: clinical and patient-oriented outcomes." *J Clin Pharm Ther* 41 (4):403-8. doi: 10.1111/jcpt.12400.

Elewa, H., F. Jalali, N. Khudair, N. Hassaballah, O. Abdelsamad, and S. Mohammed. 2016. "Evaluation of pharmacist-based compared to doctor-based anticoagulation management in Qatar." *J Eval Clin Pract* 22 (3):433-8. doi: 10.1111/jep.12504.

Eljilany, I., F. El-Dahiyat, L. E. Curley, and Z. U. Babar. 2018. "Evaluating quantity and quality of literature focusing on health economics and pharmacoeconomics in Gulf Cooperation Council countries." *Expert Rev Pharmacoecon Outcomes Res* 18 (4):403-414. doi: 10.1080/14737167.2018.1479254.

Elkassem, W., A. Pallivalapila, M. Al Hail, L. McHattie, L. Diack, and D. Stewart. 2013. "Advancing the pharmacy practice research agenda: views and experiences of pharmacists in Qatar." *Int J Clin Pharm* 35 (5):692-6. doi: 10.1007/s11096-013-9802-z.

Ertuna, E., M. Z. Arun, S. Ay, F. O. K. Kocak, B. Gokdemir, and G. Ispirli. 2019. "Evaluation of pharmacist interventions and commonly used medications in the geriatric ward of a teaching hospital in Turkey: a retrospective study." *Clin Interv Aging* 14:587-600. doi: 10.2147/CIA.S201039.

Fahs, I. M., S. Hallit, M. K. Rahal, and D. N. Malaeb. 2018. "The Community Pharmacist's Role in Reducing Cardiovascular Risk Factors in Lebanon: A Longitudinal Study." *Med Princ Pract* 27 (6):508-514. doi: 10.1159/000490853.

Farra, A., R. Zeenny, S. Nasser, N. Asmar, A. Milane, M. Bassil, M. Haidar, M. Habre, N. Zeeni, and N. Hoffart. 2018. "Implementing an interprofessional education programme in Lebanon: overcoming challenges." *East Mediterr Health J* 24 (9):914-921. doi: 10.26719/2018.24.9.914.

Gamaoun, R. 2018. "Knowledge, awareness and acceptability of anti-HPV vaccine in the Arab states of the Middle East and North Africa Region: a systematic review." *East Mediterr Health J* 24 (6):538-548. doi: 10.26719/2018.24.6.538.

Haddad, C., R. Hallit, M. Akel, K. Honein, M. Akiki, N. Kheir, S. Obeid, and S. Hallit. 2019. "Validation of the Arabic version of the ORTO-15 questionnaire in a sample of the Lebanese population." *Eat Weight Disord*. doi: 10.1007/s40519-019-00710-y.

Haddad, C., S. Hallit, M. Salhab, A. Hajj, A. Sarkis, E. N. Ayoub, H. Jabbour, and L. R. Khabbaz. 2018. "Association Between Adherence to Statins, Illness Perception, Treatment Satisfaction, and Quality of Life among Lebanese patients." *J Cardiovasc Pharmacol Ther* 23 (5):414-422. doi: 10.1177/1074248418769635.

Hajj, A., S. Hallit, E. Ramia, P. Salameh, and Subcommittee Order of Pharmacists Scientific Committee - Medication Safety. 2018. "Medication safety knowledge, attitudes and practices among community pharmacists in Lebanon." *Curr Med Res Opin* 34 (1):149-156. doi: 10.1080/03007995.2017.1361916.

Hallit S, Sacre H, Zeenny R, Hajj A, and Salameh P. 2018. "Credentialing and Recognition of Pharmacy Specializations: The Lebanese Order of Pharmacists Initiative." *ACCP International Clinical Pharmacist* (Spring):1-2.

Hallit, S., A. Hajj, H. Sacre, R. M. Zeenny, M. Akel, G. Sili, and P. Salameh. 2019. "Emphasizing the Role of Pharmacist as a Researcher: The Lebanese Order of Pharmacists' Perspective." *J Res Pharm Pract* 8 (4):229-230. doi: 10.4103/jrpp.JRPP_19_7.

Hallit, S., A. Hajj, P. Shuhaiber, K. Iskandar, E. Ramia, H. Sacre, P. Salameh, and subcommittee Order of Pharmacists of Lebanon scientific committee-Medication safety. 2019. "Medication safety knowledge, attitude, and practice among hospital pharmacists in Lebanon." *J Eval Clin Pract* 25 (2):323-339. doi: 10.1111/jep.13082.

Hallit, S., C. Raherison, D. Malaeb, R. Hallit, N. Kheir, and P. Salameh. 2018. "The AAA Risk Factors Scale: A New Model to Screen for the Risk of Asthma, Allergic Rhinitis and Atopic Dermatitis in Children." *Med Princ Pract* 27 (5):472-480. doi: 10.1159/000490704.

Hallit, S., C. Raherison, D. Malaeb, R. Hallit, M. Waked, N. Kheir, and P. Salameh. 2019. "Development of an asthma risk factors scale (ARFS) for risk assessment asthma screening in children." *Pediatr Neonatol* 60 (2):156-165. doi: 10.1016/j.pedneo.2018.05.009.

Hallit, S., C. Raherison, M. Waked, R. Hallit, N. Layoun, and P. Salameh. 2019. "Validation of the mini pediatric asthma quality of life questionnaire and identification of risk factors affecting quality of life among Lebanese children." *J Asthma* 56 (2):200-210. doi: 10.1080/02770903.2018.1441417.

Hallit, S., C. Raherison, M. Waked, and P. Salameh. 2017. "Validation of asthma control questionnaire and risk factors affecting uncontrolled asthma among the Lebanese children's population." *Respir Med* 122:51-57. doi: 10.1016/j.rmed.2016.11.018.

Hallit, S., H. Sacre, C. Haddad, D. Malaeb, G. Al Karaki, N. Kheir, A. Hajj, R. Hallit, and P. Salameh. 2019. "Development of the Lebanese insomnia scale (LIS-18): a new scale to assess insomnia in adult patients." *BMC Psychiatry* 19 (1):421. doi: 10.1186/s12888-019-2406-y.

Hallit, S., H. Sacre, A. Hajj, G. Sili, R. M. Zeenny, and P. Salameh. 2019. "Projecting the future size of the Lebanese pharmacy workforce:

forecasts until the year 2050." *Int J Pharm Pract* 27 (6):582-588. doi: 10.1111/ijpp.12564.

Hallit, S., H. Sacre, and P. Salameh. 2019. "Role of a professional organization in promoting and conducting research: the Lebanese Order of Pharmacists' experience." *Int J Pharm Pract* 27 (3):330-331. doi: 10.1111/ijpp.12517.

Hallit, S., H. Sacre, H. Sarkis, N. Dalloul, C. A. Jaoude, Z. Nahhas, J. Dagher, G. Sili, and P. Salameh. 2019. "Good Pharmacy Practice Standardized for Community Pharmacists: The Lebanese Order of Pharmacists Initiative." *J Res Pharm Pract* 8 (1):29-32. doi: 10.4103/jrpp.JRPP_18_96.

Hallit, S., R. M. Zeenny, G. Sili, and P. Salameh. 2017. "Situation analysis of community pharmacy owners in Lebanon." *Pharm Pract (Granada)* 15 (1):853. doi: 10.18549/PharmPract.2017.01.853.

Hammad, E. A., E. Elayeh, R. Tubeileh, M. Watson, and M. Wazaify. 2018. "A simulated patient study assessing over the counter supply and counseling in Jordan: responding to headache complaints." *Int J Clin Pharm* 40 (5):982-986. doi: 10.1007/s11096-018-0679-8.

Hammad, Mohamed Anwar, Khaled Mohamed Al Akhali, and Yasmin Elsobky. "A Cross-Sectional Study on Board Certified Pharmacists in Arab Countries 2018 Update." *International Journal of Humanities and Social Sciences* 14 (1):35-44.

Hammoudi, B. M., S. Ismaile, and O. Abu Yahya. 2018. "Factors associated with medication administration errors and why nurses fail to report them." *Scand J Caring Sci* 32 (3):1038-1046. doi: 10.1111/scs.12546.

Hasan, S., K. Stewart, C. B. Chapman, and D. C. M. Kong. 2018. "Physicians' perspectives of pharmacist-physician collaboration in the United Arab Emirates: Findings from an exploratory study." *J Interprof Care* 32 (5):566-574. doi: 10.1080/13561820.2018.1452726.

Haydar, S. M., S. R. Hallit, R. R. Hallit, P. R. Salameh, L. J. Faddoul, B. A. Chahine, and D. N. Malaeb. 2019. "Adherence to international guidelines for the treatment of meningitis infections in Lebanon." *Saudi Med J* 40 (3):260-265. doi: 10.15537/smj.2019.3.23965.

Hijazi, S. M., M. A. Fawzi, F. M. Ali, and K. H. Abd El Galil. 2016. "Multidrug-resistant ESBL-producing Enterobacteriaceae and associated risk factors in community infants in Lebanon." *J Infect Dev Ctries* 10 (9):947-955. doi: 10.3855/jidc.7593.

Hobeika, E., J. Farhat, J. Saab, W. Hleihel, S. Azzi-Achkouty, G. Sili, S. Hallit, and P. Salameh. 2020. "Are antibiotics substandard in Lebanon? Quantification of active pharmaceutical ingredients between brand and generics of selected antibiotics." *BMC Pharmacol Toxicol* 21 (1):15. doi: 10.1186/s40360-020-0390-y.

Huang, C. Y., S. Y. Yang, R. Mojtabai, S. K. Lin, Y. L. He, M. Y. Chong, G. Ungvari, C. H. Tan, Y. T. Xiang, N. Sartorius, N. Shinfuku, and L. Y. Chen. 2018. "Trends of Polypharmacy and Prescription Patterns of Antidepressants in Asia." *J Clin Psychopharmacol* 38 (6):598-603. doi: 10.1097/JCP.0000000000000954.

Ibrahim, Y., S. M. Hussain, S. Alnasser, H. Almohandes, and I. Sarhandi. 2018. "Patterns and sociodemographic characteristics of substance abuse in Al Qassim, Saudi Arabia: a retrospective study at a psychiatric rehabilitation center." *Ann Saudi Med* 38 (5):319-325. doi: 10.5144/0256-4947.2018.319.

Iskandar, K., S. Hallit, E. B. Raad, F. Droubi, N. Layoun, and P. Salameh. 2017. "Community pharmacy in Lebanon: A societal perspective." *Pharm Pract (Granada)* 15 (2):893. doi: 10.18549/PharmPract.2017.02.893.

Jaam, M., M. A. Hadi, N. Kheir, M. I. Mohamed Ibrahim, M. I. Diab, S. A. Al-Abdulla, and A. Awaisu. 2018. "A qualitative exploration of barriers to medication adherence among patients with uncontrolled diabetes in Qatar: integrating perspectives of patients and health care providers." *Patient Prefer Adherence* 12:2205-2216. doi: 10.2147/PPA.S174652.

Jaam, M., M. I. M. Ibrahim, N. Kheir, and A. Awaisu. 2017. "Factors associated with medication adherence among patients with diabetes in the Middle East and North Africa region: A systematic mixed studies review." *Diabetes Res Clin Pract* 129:1-15. doi: 10.1016/j.diabres.2017.04.015.

Jairoun, A., N. Hassan, A. Ali, O. Jairoun, and M. Shahwan. 2019. "Knowledge, attitude and practice of antibiotic use among university students: a cross sectional study in UAE." *BMC Public Health* 19 (1):518. doi: 10.1186/s12889-019-6878-y.

Jakovljevic, M., S. Al Ahdab, M. Jurisevic, and S. Mouselli. 2018. "Antibiotic Resistance in Syria: A Local Problem Turns Into a Global Threat." *Front Public Health* 6:212. doi: 10.3389/fpubh.2018.00212.

Jebara, T., S. Cunningham, K. MacLure, A. Pallivalapila, A. Awaisu, M. Al Hail, and D. Stewart. 2019. "Key stakeholders' views on the potential implementation of pharmacist prescribing: A qualitative investigation." *Res Social Adm Pharm*. doi: 10.1016/j.sapharm.2019.06.009.

Kamel, F. O., H. A. Alwafi, M. A. Alshaghab, Z. M. Almutawa, L. A. Alshawwa, M. M. Hagras, Y. S. Park, and A. S. Tekian. 2018. "Prevalence of prescription errors in general practice in Jeddah, Saudi Arabia." *Med Teach* 40 (sup1):S22-S29. doi: 10.1080/0142159X.2018.1464648.

Karaoui, L. R., N. Chamoun, J. Fakhir, W. Abi Ghanem, S. Droubi, A. R. Diab Marzouk, N. Droubi, H. Masri, and E. Ramia. 2019. "Impact of pharmacy-led medication reconciliation on admission to internal medicine service: experience in two tertiary care teaching hospitals." *BMC Health Serv Res* 19 (1):493. doi: 10.1186/s12913-019-4323-7.

Karimian, Z., M. Kheirandish, N. Javidnikou, G. Asghari, F. Ahmadizar, and R. Dinarvand. 2018. "Medication Errors Associated With Adverse Drug Reactions in Iran (2015-2017): A P-Method Approach." *Int J Health Policy Manag* 7 (12):1090-1096. doi: 10.15171/ijhpm.2018.91.

Katoue, M. G., and J. Ker. 2018. "Implementing the medicines reconciliation tool in practice: challenges and opportunities for pharmacists in Kuwait." *Health Policy* 122 (4):404-411. doi: 10.1016/j.healthpol.2017.12.011.

Khalifeh, M. M., N. D. Moore, and P. R. Salameh. 2017. "Self-medication misuse in the Middle East: a systematic literature review." *Pharmacol Res Perspect* 5 (4). doi: 10.1002/prp2.323.

Kheir N. 2013. "An Arab pharmacy spring: taking matters in their own hands." *Int J Clin Pharm* 35 (5):665-7. doi: 10.1007/s11096-013-9808-6.

Kheir, N., M. S. Al-Ismail, and R. Al-Nakeeb. 2017. "Can Source Triangulation Be Used to Overcome Limitations of Self-Assessments? Assessing Educational Needs and Professional Competence of Pharmacists Practicing in Qatar." *J Contin Educ Health Prof* 37 (2):83-89. doi: 10.1097/CEH.0000000000000148.

Kheir, N., A. Awaisu, H. Gad, S. Elazzazy, F. Jibril, and M. Gajam. 2015. "Clinical pharmacokinetics: perceptions of hospital pharmacists in Qatar about how it was taught and how it is applied." *Int J Clin Pharm* 37 (6):1180-7. doi: 10.1007/s11096-015-0183-3.

Kheir, N., A. Awaisu, A. Radoui, A. El Badawi, L. Jean, and R. Dowse. 2014. "Development and evaluation of pictograms on medication labels for patients with limited literacy skills in a culturally diverse multiethnic population." *Res Social Adm Pharm* 10 (5):720-30. doi: 10.1016/j.sapharm.2013.11.003.

Kheir, N., M. Zaidan, H. Younes, M. El Hajj, K. Wilbur, and P. J. Jewesson. 2008. "Pharmacy education and practice in 13 Middle Eastern countries." *Am J Pharm Educ* 72 (6):133. doi: 10.5688/aj7206133.

Kheirandish, M., V. Varahrami, A. Kebriaeezade, and A. M. Cheraghali. 2018. "Impact of economic sanctions on access to noncommunicable diseases medicines in the Islamic Republic of Iran." *East Mediterr Health J* 24 (1):42-51.

Lemay, J., F. M. Alsaleh, L. Al-Buresli, M. Al-Mutairi, E. A. Abahussain, and T. Bayoud. 2018. "Reporting of Adverse Drug Reactions in Primary Care Settings in Kuwait: A Comparative Study of Physicians and Pharmacists." *Med Princ Pract* 27 (1):30-38. doi: 10.1159/000487236.

Lemay, J., M. Waheedi, S. Al-Sharqawi, and T. Bayoud. 2018. "Medication adherence in chronic illness: do beliefs about medications play a role?" *Patient Prefer Adherence* 12:1687-1698. doi: 10.2147/PPA.S169236.

Mansoori, P. 2018. "50 years of Iranian clinical, biomedical, and public health research: a bibliometric analysis of the Web of Science Core

Collection (1965-2014)." *J Glob Health* 8 (2):020701. doi: 10.7189/jogh.08.020701.

Mansoori, P., R. Majdzadeh, Z. Abdi, I. Rudan, K. Y. Chan, Chnri Health Research Priority Setting Group Iranian, M. Aarabi, E. Ahmadnezhad, S. Ahmadnia, S. Akhondzadeh, A. Azin, F. Azizi, R. Dehnavieh, H. Eini-Zinab, F. Farzadfar, M. H. Farzaei, M. Ghanei, A. Haghdoost, S. Hantoushzadeh, G. Heydari, H. Joulaei, N. Kalantari, R. Kelishadi, A. Khosravi, B. Larijani, A. H. Mahvi, A. R. M. Bavani, A. Mesdaghinia, A. Mokri, A. Montazeri, E. Mostafavi, S. A. Motevalian, K. Naddafi, S. Nikfar, S. A. Nojoumi, M. Noroozian, A. Olyaeemanesh, N. Omidvar, A. Ostadtaghizadeh, F. Pourmalek, R. Rahimi, A. Rahimi-Movaghar, A. Rashidian, E. Razaghi, H. Sadeghi-Bazargani, G. S. Zalani, H. Soori, J. S. Tabrizi, A. Vedadhir, B. Yazdizadeh, M. Yunesian, and M. Zare. 2018. "Setting research priorities to achieve long-term health targets in Iran." *J Glob Health* 8 (2):020702. doi: 10.7189/jogh.08.020702.

Maskineh, C., and S. C. Nasser. 2018. "Managed Entry Agreements for Pharmaceutical Products in Middle East and North African Countries: Payer and Manufacturer Experience and Outlook." *Value Health Reg Issues* 16:33-38. doi: 10.1016/j.vhri.2018.04.003.

Massoud, M. A., G. Chami, M. Al-Hindi, and I. Alameddine. 2016. "Assessment of Household Disposal of Pharmaceuticals in Lebanon: Management Options to Protect Water Quality and Public Health." *Environ Manage* 57 (5):1125-37. doi: 10.1007/s00267-016-0666-6.

Mehralian, G., M. Rangchian, A. Javadi, and F. Peiravian. 2014. "Investigation on barriers to pharmaceutical care in community pharmacies: a structural equation model." *Int J Clin Pharm* 36 (5):1087-94. doi: 10.1007/s11096-014-9998-6.

Mehralian, G., M. Rangchian, and H. R. Rasekh. 2014. "Client priorities and satisfaction with community pharmacies: the situation in Tehran." *Int J Clin Pharm* 36 (4):707-15. doi: 10.1007/s11096-014-9928-7.

Mitri, R. N., C. M. Boulos, and S. M. Adib. 2017. "Aging gracefully in Greater Beirut: are there any gender-based differences?" *Eur J Public Health* 27 (3):575-581. doi: 10.1093/eurpub/ckw117.

Moghadam, Mohamad Javad Foroughi, Farzad Peiravian, Azadeh Naderi, Ali Rajabzadeh, and Hamid Reza Rasekh. 2014. "An analysis of job satisfaction among Iranian pharmacists through various job characteristics." *Iranian journal of pharmaceutical research: IJPR* 13 (3):1087.

Mokdad, A. H., M. H. Forouzanfar, F. Daoud, C. El Bcheraoui, M. Moradi-Lakeh, I. Khalil, A. Afshin, M. Tuffaha, R. Charara, R. M. Barber, J. Wagner, K. Cercy, H. Kravitz, M. M. Coates, M. Robinson, K. Estep, C. Steiner, S. Jaber, A. A. Mokdad, K. F. O'Rourke, A. Chew, P. Kim, M. M. El Razek, S. Abdalla, F. Abd-Allah, J. P. Abraham, L. J. Abu-Raddad, N. M. Abu-Rmeileh, A. A. Al-Nehmi, A. S. Akanda, H. Al Ahmadi, M. J. Al Khabouri, F. H. Al Lami, Z. A. Al Rayess, D. Alasfoor, F. S. AlBuhairan, S. F. Aldhahri, S. Alghnam, S. Alhabib, N. Al-Hamad, R. Ali, S. D. Ali, M. Alkhateeb, M. A. AlMazroa, M. A. Alomari, R. Al-Raddadi, U. Alsharif, N. Al-Sheyab, S. Alsowaidi, M. Al-Thani, K. A. Altirkawi, A. T. Amare, H. Amini, W. Ammar, P. Anwari, H. Asayesh, R. Asghar, A. M. Assabri, R. Assadi, U. Bacha, A. Badawi, T. Bakfalouni, M. O. Basulaiman, S. Bazargan-Hejazi, N. Bedi, A. R. Bhakta, Z. A. Bhutta, A. A. Bin Abdulhak, S. Boufous, R. R. Bourne, H. Danawi, J. Das, A. Deribew, E. L. Ding, A. M. Durrani, Y. Elshrek, M. E. Ibrahim, B. Eshrati, A. Esteghamati, I. A. Faghmous, F. Farzadfar, A. B. Feigl, S. M. Fereshtehnejad, I. Filip, F. Fischer, F. G. Gankpe, I. Ginawi, M. D. Gishu, R. Gupta, R. M. Habash, N. Hafezi-Nejad, R. R. Hamadeh, H. Hamdouni, S. Hamidi, H. L. Harb, M. S. Hassanvand, M. T. Hedayati, P. Heydarpour, M. Hsairi, A. Husseini, N. Jahanmehr, V. Jha, J. B. Jonas, N. E. Karam, A. Kasaeian, N. A. Kassa, A. Kaul, Y. Khader, S. E. Khalifa, E. A. Khan, G. Khan, T. Khoja, A. Khosravi, Y. Kinfu, B. K. Defo, A. L. Balaji, R. Lunevicius, C. M. Obermeyer, R. Malekzadeh, M. Mansourian, W. Marcenes, H. M. Farid, A. Mehari, A. Mehio-Sibai, Z. A. Memish, G. A. Mensah, K. A. Mohammad, Z. Nahas, J. T. Nasher, H. Nawaz, C. Nejjari, M. I. Nisar, S. B. Omer, M. Parsaeian, E. K. Peprah, A. Pervaiz, F. Pourmalek, D. M. Qato, M. Qorbani, A. Radfar, A. Rafay, K. Rahimi, V. Rahimi-Movaghar, S. U. Rahman, R. K. Rai, S. M.

Rana, S. R. Rao, A. H. Refaat, S. Resnikoff, G. Roshandel, G. Saade, M. Y. Saeedi, M. A. Sahraian, S. Saleh, L. Sanchez-Riera, M. Satpathy, S. G. Sepanlou, T. Setegn, A. Shaheen, S. Shahraz, S. Sheikhbahaei, K. Shishani, K. Sliwa, M. Tavakkoli, A. S. Terkawi, O. A. Uthman, R. Westerman, M. Z. Younis, M. El Sayed Zaki, F. Zannad, G. A. Roth, H. Wang, M. Naghavi, T. Vos, A. A. Al Rabeeah, A. D. Lopez, and C. J. Murray. 2016. "Health in times of uncertainty in the eastern Mediterranean region, 1990-2013: a systematic analysis for the Global Burden of Disease Study 2013." *Lancet Glob Health* 4 (10):e704-13. doi: 10.1016/S2214-109X(16)30168-1.

Mokdad, A. H., S. Jaber, M. I. Aziz, F. AlBuhairan, A. AlGhaithi, N. M. AlHamad, S. N. Al-Hooti, A. Al-Jasari, M. A. AlMazroa, A. M. AlQasmi, S. Alsowaidi, M. Asad, C. Atkinson, A. Badawi, T. Bakfalouni, A. Barkia, S. Biryukov, C. El Bcheraoui, F. Daoud, M. H. Forouzanfar, D. Gonzalez-Medina, R. R. Hamadeh, M. Hsairi, S. S. Hussein, N. Karam, S. E. Khalifa, T. A. Khoja, F. Lami, K. Leach-Kemon, Z. A. Memish, A. A. Mokdad, M. Naghavi, J. Nasher, M. B. Qasem, M. Shuaib, A. A. Al Thani, M. H. Al Thani, M. Zamakhshary, A. D. Lopez, and C. J. Murray. 2014. "The state of health in the Arab world, 1990-2010: an analysis of the burden of diseases, injuries, and risk factors." *Lancet* 383 (9914):309-20. doi: 10.1016/S0140-6736(13)62189-3.

Mortazavi, S. S., M. Shati, H. R. Khankeh, F. Ahmadi, S. Mehravaran, and S. K. Malakouti. 2017. "Self-medication among the elderly in Iran: a content analysis study." *BMC Geriatr* 17 (1):198. doi: 10.1186/s12877-017-0596-z.

Mourad, D., A. Hajj, S. Hallit, M. Ghossoub, and L. R. Khabbaz. 2019. "Validation of the Arabic Version of the Migraine Disability Assessment Scale Among Lebanese Patients with Migraine." *J Oral Facial Pain Headache* 33 (1):47-53. doi: 10.11607/ofph.2102.

Mukattash, T. L., M. Alattar, R. K. Abu-Farha, M. Alsous, A. S. Jarab, F. W. Darwish Elhajji, and I. L. Mukattash. 2017. "Evaluating Scientific Research Knowledge and Attitude Among Medical Representatives in

Jordan: A Cross-sectional Survey." *Curr Clin Pharmacol* 12 (4):245-252. doi: 10.2174/1574884712666170828124950.

Mukattash, T. L., A. S. Jarab, R. K. Abu-Farha, E. Alefishat, and J. C. McElnay. 2018. "Pharmaceutical Care in Children: Self-reported knowledge, attitudes and competency of final-year pharmacy students in Jordan." *Sultan Qaboos Univ Med J* 18 (4):e468-e475. doi: 10.18295/squmj.2018.18.04.007.

Naser, A. Y., I. C. K. Wong, C. Whittlesea, M. Y. Beykloo, K. K. C. Man, W. C. Y. Lau, D. A. Hyassat, and L. Wei. 2018. "Use of multiple antidiabetic medications in patients with diabetes and its association with hypoglycaemic events: a case-crossover study in Jordan." *BMJ Open* 8 (11):e024909. doi: 10.1136/bmjopen-2018-024909.

Nasr, Z. G., A. Higazy, and K. Wilbur. 2019. "Exploring the gaps between education and pharmacy practice on antimicrobial stewardship: a qualitative study among pharmacists in Qatar [Corrigendum]." *Adv Med Educ Pract* 10:307. doi: 10.2147/AMEP.S215120.

Nasr, Z. G., and K. J. Wilby. 2017. "Introducing problem-based learning into a Canadian-accredited Middle Eastern educational setting." *Curr Pharm Teach Learn* 9 (4):719-722. doi: 10.1016/j.cptl.2017.03.027.

Nazer, L. H., M. Elaibaid, N. Al-Qadheeb, R. Kleinpell, K. M. Olsen, and F. Hawari. 2018. "Critical care research in the World Health Organization Eastern Mediterranean Region over two decades: where do we stand?" *Intensive Care Med* 44 (9):1588-1590. doi: 10.1007/s00134-018-5287-5.

Paravattil, B., N. El Sakrmy, and S. Shaar. 2018. "Assessing the evidence based medicine educational needs of community pharmacy preceptors within an experiential program in Qatar." *Curr Pharm Teach Learn* 10 (1):47-53. doi: 10.1016/j.cptl.2017.09.005.

Paravattil, B., N. Kheir, and A. Yousif. 2017. "Utilization of simulated patients to assess diabetes and asthma counseling practices among community pharmacists in Qatar." *Int J Clin Pharm* 39 (4):759-768. doi: 10.1007/s11096-017-0469-8.

Pawluk, S., M. Jaam, F. Hazi, M. S. Al Hail, W. El Kassem, H. Khalifa, B. Thomas, and P. Abdul Rouf. 2017. "A description of medication errors reported by pharmacists in a neonatal intensive care unit." *Int J Clin Pharm* 39 (1):88-94. doi: 10.1007/s11096-016-0399-x.

Radi, R., U. Isleem, L. Al Omari, O. Alimoglu, H. Ankarali, and H. Taha. 2018. "Attitudes and barriers towards using complementary and alternative medicine among university students in Jordan." *Complement Ther Med* 41:175-179. doi: 10.1016/j.ctim.2018.09.012.

Rahimi, F., H. R. Rasekh, E. Abbasian, and F. Peiravian. 2018. "A new approach to pharmaceutical pricing based on patients' willingness to pay." *Trop Med Int Health* 23 (12):1326-1331. doi: 10.1111/tmi.13157.

Ramia, E., R. M. Zeenny, S. Hallit, P. Salameh, and Subcommittee Order of Pharmacists Scientific Committee - Medication Safety. 2017. "Assessment of patients' knowledge and practices regarding their medication use and risks in Lebanon." *Int J Clin Pharm* 39 (5):1084-1094. doi: 10.1007/s11096-017-0517-4.

Rouf, P. A., B. Thomas, W. Elkassem, A. Tarannum, D. Al Saad, M. M. Gasim, and M. Al Hail. 2018. "Knowledge and practice characteristics of pharmacists in Qatar towards medication use in pregnancy: a cross-sectional survey." *East Mediterr Health J* 24 (2):137-145.

Rutherford, S., and S. Saleh. 2019. "Rebuilding health post-conflict: case studies, reflections and a revised framework." *Health Policy Plan* 34 (3):230-245. doi: 10.1093/heapol/czz018.

Saade, S., S. Hallit, C. Haddad, R. Hallit, M. Akel, K. Honein, M. Akiki, N. Kheir, and S. Obeid. 2019. "Factors associated with restrained eating and validation of the Arabic version of the restrained eating scale among an adult representative sample of the Lebanese population: a cross-sectional study." *J Eat Disord* 7:24. doi: 10.1186/s40337-019-0254-2.

Sacre, H., S. Hallit, A. Hajj, R. M. Zeenny, G. Sili, and P. Salameh. 2019. "The Pharmacy Profession in a Developing Country: Challenges and Suggested Governance Solutions in Lebanon." *J Res Pharm Pract* 8 (2):39-44. doi: 10.4103/jrpp.JRPP_19_5.

Sacre, H., S. Obeid, G. Choueiry, E. Hobeika, R. Farah, A. Hajj, M. Akel, S. Hallit, and P. Salameh. 2019. "Factors associated with quality of life among community pharmacists in Lebanon: results of a cross-sectional study." *Pharm Pract (Granada)* 17 (4):1613. doi: 10.18549/PharmPract.2019.4.1613.

Sacre, H., S. Tawil, S. Hallit, A. Hajj, G. Sili, and P. Salameh. 2019. "Attitudes of Lebanese pharmacists towards online and live continuing education sessions." *Pharm Pract (Granada)* 17 (2):1438. doi: 10.18549/PharmPract.2019.2.1438.

Sacre, H., S. Tawil, S. Hallit, G. Sili, and P. Salameh. 2019. "Mandatory continuing education for pharmacists in a developing country: assessment of a three-year cycle." *Pharm Pract (Granada)* 17 (3):1545. doi: 10.18549/PharmPract.2019.3.1545.

Sakeena, M. H. F., A. A. Bennett, and A. J. McLachlan. 2018. "Non-prescription sales of antimicrobial agents at community pharmacies in developing countries: a systematic review." *Int J Antimicrob Agents* 52 (6):771-782. doi: 10.1016/j.ijantimicag.2018.09.022.

Sakr, S., S. Hallit, M. Haddad, and L. R. Khabbaz. 2018. "Assessment of potentially inappropriate medications in elderly according to Beers 2015 and STOPP criteria and their association with treatment satisfaction." *Arch Gerontol Geriatr* 78:132-138. doi: 10.1016/j.archger.2018.06.009.

Salameh, P, M Najjar Aad, M Semaan, R El Hawzi, M Bechara, B El Kadi, and L Bou Tanios. 2007. "Le circuit du médicament dans les hôpitaux libanais." ["The drug circuit in Lebanese hospitals."] *Revue d'épidémiologie et de santé publique* 55 (4):308-313.

Saleh, S., C. Abou Samra, S. Jleilaty, J. Constantin, N. El Arnaout, H. Dimassi, and D. Al-Bittar. 2017. "Perceptions and behaviors of patients and pharmacists towards generic drug substitution in Lebanon." *Int J Clin Pharm* 39 (5):1101-1109. doi: 10.1007/s11096-017-0509-4.

Saleh, S., M. Alameddine, A. Farah, N. El Arnaout, H. Dimassi, C. Muntaner, and C. El Morr. 2018. "eHealth as a facilitator of equitable access to primary healthcare: the case of caring for non-communicable diseases in rural and refugee settings in Lebanon." *Int J Public Health* 63 (5):577-588. doi: 10.1007/s00038-018-1092-8.

Sales, I., M. A. Mahmoud, H. Aljadhey, and N. I. Almeshal. 2019. "A Qualitative Approach to Improving Advanced Pharmacy Practice Experiences in an ACPE International Certified Program." *Am J Pharm Educ* 83 (2):6528. doi: 10.5688/ajpe6528.

Sam, Aaseer Thamby, and Subramani Parasuraman. 2015. "The nine-star pharmacist: An overview." *Journal of Young pharmacists* 7 (4):281.

Shawahna, R., A. Haddad, B. Khawaja, R. Raie, S. Zaneen, and T. Edais. 2016. "Medication dispensing errors in Palestinian community pharmacy practice: a formal consensus using the Delphi technique." *Int J Clin Pharm* 38 (5):1112-23. doi: 10.1007/s11096-016-0338-x.

Sheikh, J. I., S. Cheema, K. Chaabna, A. B. Lowenfels, and R. Mamtani. 2019. "Capacity building in health care professions within the Gulf cooperation council countries: paving the way forward." *BMC Med Educ* 19 (1):83. doi: 10.1186/s12909-019-1513-2.

Shilbayeh, S. A. R., W. A. Almutairi, S. A. Alyahya, N. H. Alshammari, E. Shaheen, and A. Adam. 2018. "Validation of knowledge and adherence assessment tools among patients on warfarin therapy in a Saudi hospital anticoagulant clinic." *Int J Clin Pharm* 40 (1):56-66. doi: 10.1007/s11096-017-0569-5.

Shilbayeh, S. A. R., S. A. Alyahya, N. H. Alshammari, W. A. Almutairi, and E. Shaheen. 2018. "Treatment Satisfaction Questionnaire for Medication: Validation of the Translated Arabic Version among Patients Undergoing Warfarin Therapy in Saudi Arabia." *Value Health Reg Issues* 16:14-21. doi: 10.1016/j.vhri.2018.01.007.

Sholy, L., P. Gard, S. Williams, and A. MacAdam. 2018. "Pharmacist awareness and views towards counterfeit medicine in Lebanon." *Int J Pharm Pract* 26 (3):273-280. doi: 10.1111/ijpp.12388.

Shraim, N. Y., T. A. Al Taha, R. F. Qawasmeh, H. N. Jarrar, M. A. N. Shtaya, L. A. Shayeb, and W. M. Sweileh. 2017. "Knowledge, attitudes and practices of community pharmacists on generic medicines in Palestine: a cross-sectional study." *BMC Health Serv Res* 17 (1):847. doi: 10.1186/s12913-017-2813-z.

Siddiqua, A., W. Kareem Abdul, S. Ayan, L. Al Azm, and S. Ali. 2018. "Antecedents of patients' trust in pharmacists: empirical investigation in the United Arab Emirates." *Int J Pharm Pract* 26 (1):63-72. doi: 10.1111/ijpp.12359.

Sobh, Ahmed Hesham, Zubin Austin, Mohamed Izham MI, Mohammad I Diab, and Kyle John Wilby. 2017. "Application of a systematic approach to evaluating psychometric properties of a cumulative exit-from-degree objective structured clinical examination (OSCE)." *Currents in Pharmacy Teaching and Learning* 9 (6):1091-1098.

Stewart, D., M. Al Hail, P. V. Abdul Rouf, W. El Kassem, L. Diack, B. Thomas, and A. Awaisu. 2015. "Building hospital pharmacy practice research capacity in Qatar: a cross-sectional survey of hospital pharmacists." *Int J Clin Pharm* 37 (3):511-21. doi: 10.1007/s11096-015-0087-2.

Stewart, D., B. Thomas, K. MacLure, A. Pallivalapila, W. El Kassem, A. Awaisu, J. S. McLay, K. Wilbur, K. Wilby, C. Ryan, A. Dijkstra, R. Singh, and M. Al Hail. 2018. "Perspectives of healthcare professionals in Qatar on causes of medication errors: A mixed methods study of safety culture." *PLoS One* 13 (9):e0204801. doi: 10.1371/journal.pone.0204801.

Stewart, D., B. Thomas, K. MacLure, K. Wilbur, K. Wilby, A. Pallivalapila, A. Dijkstra, C. Ryan, W. El Kassem, A. Awaisu, J. S. McLay, R. Singh, and M. Al Hail. 2018. "Exploring facilitators and barriers to medication error reporting among healthcare professionals in Qatar using the theoretical domains framework: A mixed-methods approach." *PLoS One* 13 (10):e0204987. doi: 10.1371/journal.pone.0204987.

Thamby S. A., and Parasuraman S. 2015. "The nine-star pharmacist: An overview." *Journal of Young pharmacists* 7 (4):281.

Thomas, B., V. Paudyal, K. MacLure, A. Pallivalapila, J. McLay, W. El Kassem, M. Al Hail, and D. Stewart. 2019. "Medication errors in hospitals in the Middle East: a systematic review of prevalence, nature, severity and contributory factors." *Eur J Clin Pharmacol* 75 (9):1269-1282. doi: 10.1007/s00228-019-02689-y.

Wilbur, K. 2013. "Pharmacovigilance in the Middle East: a survey of 13 arabic-speaking countries." *Drug Saf* 36 (1):25-30. doi: 10.1007/s40264-012-0001-y.

Wilbur, K., and A. D. J. Taylor. 2018. "Does a blended learning environment suit advanced practice training for pharmacists in a Middle East setting?" *Int J Pharm Pract* 26 (6):560-567. doi: 10.1111/ijpp.12437.

Wilby, K. J., and M. Diab. 2016. "Key challenges for implementing a Canadian-based objective structured clinical examination (OSCE) in a Middle Eastern context." *Can Med Educ J* 7 (3):e4-e9.

Wilby, K. J., M. Zolezzi, O. Rachid, and A. El-Kadi. 2017. "Development of a college-level assessment framework in line with international accreditation standards: A Middle Eastern perspective." *Curr Pharm Teach Learn* 9 (1):115-120. doi: 10.1016/j.cptl.2016.08.028.

Yaacoub, S. G., N. A. Lahoud, N. J. Francis, D. W. Rahme, T. H. Murr, P. F. Maison, and N. G. Saleh. 2019. "Antibiotic Prescribing Rate in Lebanese Community Pharmacies: A Nationwide Patient-Simulated Study of Acute Bacterial Rhinosinusitis." *J Epidemiol Glob Health* 9 (1):44-49. doi: 10.2991/jegh.k.190305.001.

Yaghoubifard, S., A. Rashidian, A. Kebriaeezadeh, R. Majdzadeh, S. A. Hosseini, A. Akbari Sari, and J. Salamzadeh. 2015. "Developing a conceptual framework and a tool for measuring access to, and use of, medicines at household level (HH-ATM tool)." *Public Health* 129 (5):444-52. doi: 10.1016/j.puhe.2015.01.026.

Yousuf, S. A., M. Alshakka, W. F. S. Badulla, H. S. Ali, P. R. Shankar, and M. I. Mohamed Ibrahim. 2019. "Attitudes and practices of community pharmacists and barriers to their participation in public health activities in Yemen: mind the gap." *BMC Health Serv Res* 19 (1):304. doi: 10.1186/s12913-019-4133-y.

Yusuff, K. B. 2015. "Does self-reflection and peer-assessment improve Saudi pharmacy students' academic performance and metacognitive skills?" *Saudi Pharm J* 23 (3):266-75. doi: 10.1016/j.jsps.2014.11.018.

Zakaria, N., O. AlFakhry, A. Matbuli, A. Alzahrani, N. S. S. Arab, A. Madani, N. Alshehri, and A. I. Albarrak. 2018. "Development of Saudi e-health literacy scale for chronic diseases in Saudi Arabia: using integrated health literacy dimensions." *Int J Qual Health Care* 30 (4):321-328. doi: 10.1093/intqhc/mzy033.

Zeenny, R., S. Wakim, and Y. M. Kuyumjian. 2017. "Potentially inappropriate medications use in community-based aged patients: a cross-sectional study using 2012 Beers criteria." *Clin Interv Aging* 12:65-73. doi: 10.2147/CIA.S87564.

Zeidan, R. K., C. Haddad, R. Hallit, M. Akel, K. Honein, M. Akiki, N. Kheir, S. Hallit, and S. Obeid. 2019. "Validation of the Arabic version of the binge eating scale and correlates of binge eating disorder among a sample of the Lebanese population." *J Eat Disord* 7:40. doi: 10.1186/s40337-019-0270-2.

Zeidan, R. K., S. Hallit, R. M. Zeenny, and P. Salameh. 2019. "Lebanese community-based pharmacists' interest, practice, knowledge, and barriers towards pharmacy practice research: A cross-sectional study." *Saudi Pharm J* 27 (4):550-557. doi: 10.1016/j.jsps.2019.02.002.

Zolezzi, M., O. Abdallah, N. Kheir, and A. G. Abdelsalam. 2019. "Evaluation of community pharmacists' preparedness for the provision of cardiovascular disease risk assessment and management services: A study with simulated patients." *Res Social Adm Pharm* 15 (3):252-259. doi: 10.1016/j.sapharm.2018.04.032.

Zolezzi, M., C. A. Sadowski, N. Al-Hasan, and O. Gad Alla. 2018. "Geriatric education in schools of pharmacy: Students' and educators' perspectives in Qatar and Canada." *Curr Pharm Teach Learn* 10 (9):1184-1196. doi: 10.1016/j.cptl.2018.06.010.

In: Pharmacists
Editor: Line L. Villadsen

ISBN: 978-1-53618-018-3
© 2020 Nova Science Publishers, Inc.

Chapter 4

PHARMACISTS IN LOW- AND MIDDLE-INCOME COUNTRIES: CHALLENGES AND PERSPECTIVES

Thang Nguyen[1,], Linh T. K. Mai[1], Vu T. Nguyen[1], Thu T. A. Truong[1], Tu T. C. Le[1], Suol T. Pham[1], Chu X. Duong[1], Thao H. Nguyen[2], Susan E. Matthews[3] and Katja Taxis[4]*

[1]Department of Pharmacology and Clinical Pharmacy,
Can Tho University of Medicine and Pharmacy, Can Tho, Vietnam
[2]Department of Clinical Pharmacy,
University of Medicine and Pharmacy at Ho Chi Minh City,
Ho Chi Minh City, Vietnam
[3]School of Pharmacy, University of East Anglia,
Norwich, The U.K.
[4]Unit of PharmacoTherapy, Epidemiology & Economics,
Groningen Research Institute of Pharmacy, University of Groningen,
Groningen, The Netherlands

---

[*] Corresponding Author's Email: nthang@ctump.edu.vn.

ABSTRACT

Over the last decades, there have been several changes in the pharmacist's role in the primary care system due to the esatblishment of clinical pharmacy and community pharmacy. Their contribution to the translation of evidence-based knowledge into clinical practice is helpful in the optimisation of the use of drugs. For example, pharmacists provide recommendations to both medical staff and society in the treatment and prevention of diseases. They are not only responsible for preventing medication errors and solving drug-problems but also providing pharmaceutical care services, especially in chronic disorders. However, in low- and middle- income countries, this clinical practice is a very new area and pharmacists face many social barriers to improve their role. The awareness of the community about the pharmacist's role is still limited and there are many conflicts between pharmacists and other medical staff. Lack of human resources and investments are also challenging for developing the role of clinical and community pharmacists. Raising the knowledge of citizens and developing a way to cope with these barriers is essential to developing the pharmacists' roles as a major part of the medical team and provide patients with the highest outcomes and lowest cost.

Keywords: clinical pharmacy, community pharmacy, chronic diseases, pharmaceutical care, low- and middle-income countries, patient outcomes

1. THE ROLE OF PHARMACIST: PAST AND PRESENT

Nowadays people live in a modern society which has a high quality of healthcare services. Along with the advancement of the healthcare system, it is undeniable that the role of pharmacists has changed dramatically and reached a high level in a variety of pharmaceutical and clinical areas. Thus, pharmacists not only engage in drug manufacturing and supply but also provide patients with many health services to optimize their treatment [1].

The profession of pharmacy has been established for a long time, since leaves were first used on wounds to reduce physical pain. Many records provide evidence that in ancient Babylon, Egypt, pharmacists played a role as of the *"apothecary"* (a person who prepared and sold medicines and drugs). Medicine and pharmacy were developed together as a whole until the 13th century in Europe. While there was a distinction between them, pharmacists only did the job as an apothecary and drug-seller until the industrial revolution when they also took a role in manufacturing and research for new drugs [2].

With the significant growth in available drugs came difficulties for both clinicians and patients in using them for treatment and the establishment of the role of hospital pharmacist; the first recorded American hospital pharmacist was Jonathan Roberts in 1752. A few years later, there was a wider role of pharmacists in hospitals supporting clinicians to improve patient outcomes. Adverse drug reaction (ADR) identification and management is a good example. Since the 1960s, the *"thalidomide disaster"* with the phocomelia of an absence of limbs in babies has made the medical profession pay significant attention to the side effects of drugs and increased the role of pharmacists in ADR monitoring and other clinical impacts [3].

Because of this awareness, the education of specialist pharmacists suitable to work in hospitals was developed. Thanks to the formation of *Doctor of Pharmacy degree programs*, the first generation of American pharmacists graduated in the 1950s that were able to support clinicians in pharmacotherapy for patients with chronic diseases such as hypertension. It was described firstly and published in the cardiology journal *Circulation* in 1973. Moreover, the pharmacists who are responsible for patient care were then classified into two popular fields: *dispensing pharmacy* (community pharmacy) and *direct patient care* (included clinical pharmacy and ambulatory care). Since this period, a new view of citizens about pharmacists' roles has been formed. In the 1980s, clinical pharmacists in many developed countries began to focus on especially unique areas such as cardiology, oncology, infectious disease, etc. By providing clinicians and patients with essential drug information and suggesting to them the best choice of medication, the role of pharmacists was gradually improved. It thus led to the establishment of a new concept, *Pharmaceutical care* which strongly highlights the responsibility of the pharmacist to work directly with the patient to optimize their treatment processes. Nowadays, while the indispensable role of pharmacists in developed countries has been shown

[4], the popular perception regarding the contribution of pharmacists in low- and middle-income countries (LMICs) has been limited to a focus on supplying and manufacturing generic products. These countries have developed clinical pharmacy programs much later, in the 1990s or after. For example, it was added to the pharmacist's curriculum of Vietnam and India respectively in 1993 and 1996. This text will show how the pharmacist contributes to improving patient outcomes in the healthcare system, the barrier of their development in LMICs and many feasible solutions for these problems [5].

2. THE BASIC DEFINITION OF A PATIENT-CARING PHARMACIST

In the 20th century, pharmacists in hospitals began their role as a member of the interprofessional patient care team to provide healthcare services to patients to optimize their medication-related outcomes. This resulted in the creation of *clinical pharmacists* [1] who are responsible for services such as drug information, drug order fulfilment and patient education.

It is clear that *clinical pharmacists* provide *direct patient care* within their role. According to ACCP, this means "the direct observation and evaluation of the patient and his/her medication-related needs; the initiation, modification, or discontinuation of patient-specific pharmacotherapy; and the ongoing pharmacotherapeutic monitoring and follow-up of patients in collaboration with other health professionals" [6]. In other words, this definition established significantly wider assignments of pharmacists in the healthcare system than traditionally.

While *clinical pharmacists* work in the hospital, others do their job by providing primary care services at patient's homes known as *ambulatory care*. These services have gained popularity with elderly patients in developed countries as America and Canada. Both clinical pharmacists and those providing ambulatory care have a direct impact on patients. And thus, they provide *pharmaceutical care*. The concepts of *pharmaceutical care* were formed in the final years of the last century. According to Hepler and Strand (1989), it is the responsible provision of *pharmacotherapy* for the purpose of a definite outcome that improves a patient's quality of life. It strongly appreciates the relationship between patients and the clinical pharmacists [7].

Additionally, *community pharmacy* or *retail pharmacy* is another health care occupation in which the pharmacist can directly interact with patients in their drugstores or community health centers. As well as clinical pharmacists, the pharmacists in community with these responsibilities, not only prepare and dispense many kinds of drugs but also guarantee the accuracy and safety of the prescription and educate the patients in using drugs to optimize their outcomes. They maintain links with other health professionals to play their role in primary care [1].

3. THE IMPACT OF PHARMACISTS ON IMPROVING HEALTHCARE QUALITY

3.1. Drug Information

Drug information (DI) is one of the main services provided by the pharmacist in hospital and community pharmacy. They offer advice about medicines and their role in disease management to the patients, physicians and general population. While medical science nowadays develops with a rapid rate, the number of new drugs and associated information is rising significantly too. The advances, unfortunately, create an information gap for health professionals and patients resulting in uninformed choices of pharmacotherapy. Therefore, DI services are pivotal today to deliver evidence-based and timely critical information either orally or written. In developing countries, the activities undertaken by DI pharmacists are the same as everywhere; answering questions related to drugs, writing bulletins, participating in medical workshops, performing pharmacovigilance, and providing training related to drug information. As a result, DI pharmacists can contribute dramatically to alleviating worldwide problems of safe and effective use of medications [8, 9].

3.2. ADRs Reports and Pharmacovigilance

Besides DI services, it is essential to collect and analyse reports of adverse drug reactions (ADRs) in clinical treatment. The majority of proven side effects in the summary of product characteristics (SPCs) are discovered in controlled conditions with selected patients. However potential risks, caused by the active element, excipients or even impurities formed in the storage process are more likely to be observed after regulation. Reactions can affect patients with a wide range of levels, from slight to serious, and some are unpredictable in the early stages such as *hypomagnesaemia* caused by *bevacizumab*. Even in developed countries, ADR related deaths are a matter of serious concern, so it is necessary for clinical and community pharmacists to continually observe, identify and manage the risks of ADRs. Furthermore, it has been suggested that collaboration between academia, health care providers including a pharmacist, patient, manufacturer, government, media, and civil society in building a *pharmacovigilance system* should be improved, especially in developing countries where there is a lack of this close-knit relationship [10, 11].

3.3. Medication Safety Improvements

3.3.1. Medication Errors

On the other hand, medication safety risk is one of the most important factors jeopardizing patients. There are a number of issues relating to medication safety including medication error (ME), drug interactions in prescription, etc. ME in recent years has caused a high rate of mortality, morbidity and also raised treatment costs. The hospital pharmacist, as an active member of a healthcare team, plays a vital role in examining and assessing throughout the drug distribution chain; from prescribing, drug choice, dispensing and preparation to the administration of drugs, to ensure medication safety. For example, they can offer their interventions in the drug pathways in direct or indirect ways such as checking the patient is systematically prescribed in the hospital management software [12, 13, 14, 15].

In some developing countries, these activities have not had a high enough influence on the quality of treatment compared to developed countries. For example, despite a clinical pharmacist-led training programme on clinically relevant errors during intravenous (IV) medication preparation and administration conducted in the intensive care unit (ICU) in a *Vietnamese* hospital error rates remain relatively high, suggesting that the training programme should be improved to raise medication safety [16].

3.3.2. Drug Interaction Management

Another issue regarding medication safety is drug interactions. It is known that the elderly, who often need to use multiple drugs for long-term treatment, usually have a high risk of drug interactions, and a large proportion may be potentially harmful to their health. Take an example for this adverse effect, while patients use cimetidine, an antihistamine H2, along with warfarin, the concentrations of the oral anticoagulant may be increased leading to the risk of bleeding. The practice in clinical pharmacy also ensures that these detrimental drug interactions are minimized. By their professional knowledge, the pharmacist attempts to limit the adverse effect of drug interactions by avoiding unnecessary combinations, adjusting the doses of the required drug, spacing dosage times, providing information or educating about risk factors, etc. Drugs can interact with any substances, including foods and drinks, which should be discussed with physicians before prescribing, such as the case of *ciprofloxacin* an antibiotic agent that should not be administered at the same time as milk to avoid flexical reactions that reduce the absorption of the drug. For these reasons, most researchers agree that the pharmacist has a key role in drug interactions management to reduce the potential risk of multi-medications and optimize patient outcomes [17].

3.3.3. Interventions on Inappropriate Prescribing

The rate of inappropriate prescribing can be really high in hospitals and is the main cause of risks of adverse effects, interactions and other drug-related hospitalizations. As a pharmacotherapy expert, the pharmacist, has the knowledge and ability to identify and manage drug-related problems (DRPs) and Negative Outcomes Associated with Medications (NOMs). Checking-out drug interactions rapidly is a particular example. In many cases, the mechanisms of these interactions are flexible, such as pharmacokinetic interactions. It is clear that pharmacists can support physicians to prevent DRPs in these cases. On the other hand, they can send patients an educational prescribing brochure in parallel to giving their physicians an evidence-based pharmaceutical opinion to recommend deprescribing. As a consequence, the rate of inappropriate prescribing is reduced alongside an increase in medication adherence of patients [18, 19].

3.4. Pharmaceutical Care and Its Clinical Benefits

Pharmaceutical care, perspicuously, is a service provided by the pharmacist in hospitals or community drugstores that directly helps patients optimize their medication effects. This activity aims to achieve the best outcomes; including reducing the symptoms, delaying the chronic disease process, preventing side effects and also reducing the cost of treatment. Firstly, the role of pharmacists in pharmaceutical care is to assist the patient in their self-management which is a key approach to manage communicable diseases. For example, they can provide more information about the drug prescribed for patients and discuss with patients about the drug effects, the time to use, the adverse reactions, and then give some beneficial advice regarding medication care if the patients have difficulty taking it. In order to achieve this, collaborative care between the pharmacists and patients is especially important. Thus, establishing a familiar relationship with patients and raising their trust are vital for pharmacists [20, 21].

Nowadays, pharmacists possess pivotal skills which qualify them for playing active roles in the processes of design and application of clinical pathways (CPs). Such pathways reduce in-hospital complications, increase the rate of documentation of the staff, decline the length of stay (-2.5 days for CPs compared to -0.8 days for the standard of care) and also the cost of treatment. On the other hand, CPs provide unique opportunities for building a *patient-centered pharmaceutical model* and allowing pharmacists to demonstrate interprofessional leadership skills in multidisciplinary collaborations [22].

Pharmacists have the potential to design and follow the pharmaceutical care plans for many patients. In Canada, pharmacists have been shown to be an important member of *family medicine groups* (FMGs) e.g., in January 2019, according to the Ministry, 262 (79%) of the 333 FMGs had a working agreement with one or more pharmacists, and this proportion is continuously expanding [23].

However, in a study in Hong Kong, while pharmacists believed that they had an extended role in addition to drug management to prevent health deterioration and save healthcare cost, others argued that they were drug experts only and could only play an assisting role [20].

4. THE IMPACT OF PHARMACISTS ON CHRONIC DISEASE MANAGEMENT

4.1. Role of Pharmacist in Non-Communicable Disease Management

Diabetes and cardiovascular diseases such as hypertension, heart failure and chronic coronary disease are common non-communicable diseases which have high levels of complications leading to death in both developed and developing countries. Approximately 80% of patients with diabetes live in LMICs. Controlling blood glucose, blood pressure and LDL-cholesterol level is the best way to delay the disease process. Due to the available treatment, less than 10-20% of patients achieve this in therapy [24]. A number of studies have demonstrated the effectiveness of interventions of clinical and community pharmacists in patient outcomes. For example, it was demonstrated in the United States that pharmacist-led pharmaceutical care was effective in improving HbA1c in patients with diabetes in both LMICs and high-income countries (HIc) [25]. It was also shown that pharmacist-managed care possesses a potential role in protection from diabetes retinopathy (DR) and other complications [26]. Also, in patients with hypertension, the pharmaceutical care intervention offered by clinical pharmacists has a significant improvement in diastolic blood pressure (DBP) [27].

Regarding more serious outcomes, poor adherence to medications and other aspects of lifestyles are likely to play a significant role. In fact, management of diabetes is challenging because patients should adopt several self-care behaviors including dietary modification, physical activity, weight loss, medication adherence, and blood glucose monitoring. A community pharmacist–delivered diabetes support program in Iran has been shown to improve *medication adherence, self-care practice, and weight control* in patients [28]. Similarly, other studies have emphasized an important role for clinical pharmacists in delivering education for hypertensive patients and assisting them in taking medications [29]. Cardiovascular disease, in general, is on the rise in many developing countries and this is coupled with a lack of awareness of diseases and drug-related information [30].

According to the WHO, the economy and social conditions are just one of five factors affecting poor adherence to medications. Therefore, the cost of treatment plays a vital role in the discontinuation of drugs in patients with chronic diseases. In fact, a pharmacist can contribute to decreasing the healthcare cost burden of chronic patients. In some developing countries like Nepal, it was shown that pharmacists' intervention through a pharmaceutical care program significantly decreased direct healthcare costs of diabetics in test groups compared to control groups and minimized the healthcare cost burden of patients directly [31]. Similar studies also highlighted the cost-effectiveness of a clinical pharmacy intervention for hypertension control in primary care settings [32].

Besides cardiovascular and metabolic diseases, cancer is also a chronic non-communicable disease that has a high level of incidence around the world. Pain is one of the most common symptoms in cancer patients, which causes patients' anxiety, depression, fatigue, insomnia and loss of appetite, thus affecting their routine activities, social interactions, and quality of life. In fact, cancer pain control is a complex issue that requires collaboration of the multidisciplinary team including many health professionals such as anesthesiologists, physicians, neurologists, nurses, pharmacists, etc. Many studies have been conducted to determinate the role of pharmacists engaging in the clinical teams in oncology treatment. There are three general effects of pharmacists. Firstly, the pharmacist is considered to be an expert on drug information, especially on *opioids* and *antineoplastic drugs*. *Opioids* are indispensable analgesics widely used for the treatment of moderate-to-severe cancer pain. However, in some countries like China, opioid treatment management is poor for many reasons; many patients prefer bearing pain because they are afraid of the possibility of drug addiction while oncologists have misunderstanding of analgesics selection, administration dose and duration [33, 34].

In China, it was shown that by giving lectures or presentations on cancer pain and distributing information on analgesics pharmacists could play a role in educating patients on how to express and assess their pain and to dispel their fears and analgesic myths. In the U.S and Canada, the clinical pharmacist system is much more mature, and opioids are both frequently used and subject to national guidelines. However, in developing countries like Nepal, the importance of pharmacists is only highlighted in the preparation, dispensing, and oversight of cytotoxic drugs, although pharmaceutical care in cancer is slightly developed [35].

Secondly, pharmacists can become more competent in assessing pain intensity through clinical training programs, which is necessary for determining analgesic dosages. Particularly, the pharmacist can take advantage of the pain scale to evaluate the conditions, listen to patients and develop rapport to gain insight into their condition. After that, they can recommend rational drug use for patients including opioids, chemotherapeutic agents, adjunct medicines and also traditional Chinese herbs. As an expert in pharmacotherapy, they can assist oncologists in designing a treatment plan, not only to optimize the efficacy of cancer treatment, but also to minimize the adverse effects of drug interactions and medication errors [34, 35].

Thirdly, pharmacists' follow-up is needed to ensure the effectiveness, adherence and safety management of cancer pain control. They are responsible for keeping in touch with patients, carrying out distance medication and solving adverse drug reactions for patients. As a result of these interventions, there is a rise in the quality and standardization of cancer pain therapy [33, 34, 35].

4.2. Role of Pharmacists in Management of Infectious Diseases and Antibiotic Resistance

In the LMICs, the rate of communicable disease incidences is very high. Moreover, inappropriate and overused antimicrobial prescribing in clinical practice impacts significantly on the growth of *antibiotic resistance* (AR). The number of antibiotics that have been developed in recent years is very small making the preservation of currently available antibiotics paramount. Nowadays, it is considered a global health challenge and developing countries are more vulnerable to these adverse health impacts [36].

In many countries, *antibiotic stewardship programmes* (ASP) have been established to control antimicrobial prescribing, possibly minimizing the emergence of resistant organisms. It is believed that pharmacists as the main supplier and regulator of antibiotics can play a key role to support the appropriate use of these medicines in developing countries and reduce AR. Many studies have been conducted to identify the effect of pharmacist involvement particularly highlighting the roles that pharmacists play in maximizing the utility of available drugs by training other medical staff and managing the prescription activities. However, there is a lack of knowledge relating to infectious diseases for some clinical and community pharmacists in many hospitals and drugstores, especially in the LMICs. Therefore, continuous educational programmes should be directed to the pharmacists to promote the accurate management of patients [37, 38, 39].

Additionally, for patients with severe infections and multidrug-resistant infections, it is easy to use a dose that leads to an inadequate antimicrobial concentration at the site of infection and is associated with poor patient outcomes. As a member of the medical team, a pharmacist can also help to design an effective antimicrobial dosing regimen based on pharmacokinetic/pharmacodynamic (PK/PD) models. As some antibiotics have time-dependent effectiveness while others have concentration-dependent effectiveness, the daily-dose and dosage intervals of antibiotic must be calculated and designed appropriately to optimize the outcomes of infectious treatment. The mechanism of antibiotic action and other characteristics are the specialized knowledge of pharmacists who can support physicians and nurses in clinical practice, especially in these cases which combinations of antibiotics is necessary or there is a narrow-therapeutic range [40].

5. THE DEVELOPMENT OF THE PHARMACIST'S ROLES IN HEALTHCARE SYSTEM

5.1. The Perspectives of Patients and Other Medical Staff on the Roles of Pharmacists in the Healthcare System

Pharmacists have been known as the health care professional responsible for providing drugs to doctors and patients for a long time [41]. Recently, however, the number of tasks that are expected of them has grown, pharmacists contribute not only to the healthcare team but also more widely to the community. The role of pharmacists should be extended in the primary healthcare system [23, 42], however, in developing countries, clinical pharmacy is a very new field in pharmaceutical care. The concepts of clinical pharmacists and community pharmacists as well as their duties and skills are not clear in these countries, moreover, the community usually pays little attention to defining pharmacists and their roles [43].

5.1.1. Perspective of Patients about Pharmacists

The shortage of medical staff in Europe is expected to be continuous with the severity depending on the health system of each country. In response to this trend, the role of pharmacists in many European countries is growing towards being more patient-focused and expanding the amount of primary care available through community pharmacy. The role of "Community Pharmacist" has been defined through the theme "The Role of the Pharmacist in the Health Care System" - WHO, 1994. Pharmacy practice worldwide is evolving from dispensing and educating patients to providing patient-centered care where pharmacists asses the justifiable medication therapy, ensure patients have an understanding of their drug therapy, encourage adherence to medications, and monitor patient outcomes [36]. Communication between patients and pharmacists has been improved to be a two-way process [21]. The old way of communication was a one-way process from sender to receiver, where the pharmacist concentrated mainly on providing medical information, therefore, no response was received from patients who were not fully aware of their aspiration or adherence. The two-way process is more likely a conversation between two participants such as in patient-centered communication where the pharmacist identifies and responds to patients' comments and feelings regarding their illness. The main difference between the patient-centered and biomedical models is the level of patient engagement. Patients have more opportunity to contact with pharmacists in the newer approach and thus have a clearer vision about them and their role [42, 44, 45].

Pharmacists may be accessible to patients at times when physicians are not, especially in rural communities. In many countries, pharmacists are accepted as a reasonable alternative for seeking care from a physician. Pharmacist treatment of minor ailments and conditions has been recognized for reducing health care costs, improving access through decreasing wait times and reducing emergency department visits. Through community pharmacy, patients have more opportunities to receive the support of pharmacists. However, in LMICs, community pharmacy is still too underdeveloped to act as a main health information system for patients in an area.

Patients also require treatment services in pharmacies for minor ailments and conditions, especially when the patient is unable or unwilling to get an appointment with a physician. Community pharmacists are usually the first point of contact for patients seeking advice on common health issues [36]. However, there is a lack of community awareness that pharmacists are able to provide these services to patients and help address the gap in health care access found in rural communities in for example, the UK [46]. Patients agree that they would not be averse to accessing care provided by a pharmacist, if they knew these services were being offered. Despite the availability of training for pharmacists to provide treatment services for minor ailments and conditions, some pharmacists are still limited in their implementation because the patient prefers to access physician services [47].

Patient self-management is a key approach to managing non-communicable diseases (NCDs, e.g., cardiovascular diseases, cancer, chronic respiratory diseases and diabetes mellitus). A pharmacist-led approach in patient self-management means collaborative care between pharmacists and patients, where they make healthcare decisions together. However, the development of both patient self-management and the role of pharmacists is limited. In Nepal, pharmacists can contribute by screening and monitoring; counseling on lifestyle; providing medication therapy management services; promoting public health; and providing other pharmaceutical services [48] but pharmacists still lack training in engaging with young people. Community pharmacy staff are unsure whether their adult-focused services should be offered to young people, especially those aged <16 years. Building long-term relationships with young people was seen as a priority, especially with young patients who have chronic illnesses. It was proposed that pharmacists should have psychological counseling to share ideas about their current and future roles in the support of young people who take medication for chronic illnesses as young people may be more open to the pharmacist as a health information channel than adults. In a survey, pharmacist support of the development of generic health care skills among young people (such as getting a prescription refill and minimizing copayments) received the highest prioritization followed by developing enough specialist knowledge to ensure medication use is safe for all patients.

There are a number of medication-related problems that particularly concern young people, such as interactions of drugs and alcohol, and side effects that usually happen at young ages and pharmacists need to recognize these issues to offer relevant advice [21, 49].

On the other hand, the increase in the elderly population leads to an increase in the prevalence of diseases due to the high risk of having one or more chronic diseases. They are the largest consumer of medications and health care resources. Elderly patients visit the pharmacies regularly to refill their medications, this provides pharmacists with the opportunities to review and adjust their medications [50]. This is especially important for patients who are receiving treatment from different medical specializations which put them at higher risk of drug duplication, drug–drug interactions and adverse drug events [50, 51].

Having more forms of pharmacy interactions has improved the communication with patients to control their situation better. Several studies had been conducted to examine the engagement of pharmacists in providing pharmaceutical care to patients. Many studies showed that the involvement of pharmacists in primary healthcare increased medication appropriateness, increased patients' medication knowledge and adherence, reduced the occurrence of drug-related problems (DRPs), decreased mortality and adverse drug reactions (ADRs) [52].

5.1.2. Perspective of Other Healthcare Professionals about Pharmacists

Pharmacists, especially those working in hospitals, often collaborate with other medical staff to carry out clinical pharmacy work. They are the ones who provide colleagues accurate drug information and intervene on inappropriate medication prescribing. For a long time, nearly all physicians have been willing to collaborate with Pharmacists, but only on medication issues. Physicians would still be the ones prescribing medications while pharmacists would suggest the most appropriate medications and assist in monitoring patients' drug interactions and side-effects.

Despite undertaking a range of different activities, awareness of other medical staff on the pharmacists' role is not high because clinical pharmacy is still a new field in developing countries. In order to improve medication adherence and consequently patient outcomes, it is necessary to develop strategies to improve collaborative relationships between pharmacists and other medical staff. The majority of pharmacists in Hong Kong stated that it was necessary to collaborate with physicians, TCM practitioners, nurses, diabetic nurses, dieticians and social workers in handling chronic cases [20].

Some physicians feel that the relationship with pharmacists may not be taken seriously due to the possible effect of suspicion on patient-doctor relationship. More recently, however, the pharmacist's role has evolved into a patient-centered approach, and that has some doctors concerned about the threat to their medical professional status. Pharmacist's comments about his use of the drug may create suspicion for the patients.

Moreover, physicians who do not want to have any conflict in front of the patients want to see the patients themselves, and have more consultations by themselves, and they are afraid the pharmacist-physician relationship will affect their therapeutic results. Some physicians question the experience of pharmacists and their ability to provide comprehensive care. In their opinion, pharmacists sometimes do not have enough clinical and practical abilities needed for the evaluation of patients. Nearly all physicians were willing to collaborate with pharmacists, but only on medication issues [20].

Community pharmacists in Canada reported that the major occasions for contacting general practitioners (GPs) are for contraindications, drug interactions, and unclear prescriptions. Some participating pharmacists have had positive experiences when interacting with GPs, most claim to meet GPs periodically on phones and get answers to their queries. Most family doctors have reported on regular phone calls from the community pharmacists in the case of unreasonable prescriptions. GPs often appreciate this type of safety net. However, only some GPs have commented that they will contact the pharmacist on their own initiative. The main reason given is lack of time [23].

Instead of seeing these queries as supportive, pharmacists often have a feeling that GPs consider requests to be invasive and controlling. Some pharmacists have reported negative experiences, and disrespect when contacting a doctor. Compared to pharmacists working in cities, people working in rural and provincial areas have less negative experience when contacting family doctors. They often have long-term working experience with local physicians by mutual trust and appreciation.

This is not only the case in developing countries, in another study in Mecklenburg-Western Pomerania, a predominantly rural region of North-Eastern Germany, GPs identified themselves as the most responsible for patients taking a drug. They feel that pharmacists miss basic information about patients on their medical history and lack of expertise and knowledge to understand and refactor the doctor's theory in many cases [53].

A rewarding aspect for the pharmacists was the respect they received during one-on-one discussions and how their professional credibility shaped future interactions. Pharmacists felt a sense of pride and professional satisfaction that they were able to contribute to a medical doctor's learning with the potential of exerting a positive influence on patient care. They became cognisant of the need to listen and reflect in order to obtain information which allowed them to communicate effectively and selectively tailor the discussion topic to the individual's practice and needs.

The need for transferring information from the hospital team to the community pharmacist is also a priority. Hospital pharmacists reflected on the need for better routine communication with community pharmacy colleagues and the challenge to incorporate that into their daily activities. Furthermore, the degree of integration of pharmacists working in primary care teams with patient-centred clinical pharmacy services is associated with improved health outcomes [44]. Community pharmacists were surprised at the value and trust of physicians for them as a source of medication information. Generally, both community and health professionals had improved their awareness relating to the expanding roles of pharmacists [52].

5.2. The Challenges of Developing the Pharmacists' Role in the Healthcare System

Over the past two decades, the role of pharmacists has expanded beyond medication dispensing, packaging and compounding (WHO 1998). Pharmacists are increasingly considered part of the health care system whether in community pharmacies, primary health centers or hospitals (Ghani 2010; WHO 1998) [54]. Pharmacists are challenged, however, to become key actors in optimising and monitoring medication use and to become advocates for patients.

Pharmacists also play an important role in self-medication and self-care by providing and interpreting information regarding appropriate healthcare and medication choices and promoting the rational use of drugs. Furthermore, the significant increase in health demand leading to complex medication uses, and poor adherence of patients has provided additional opportunities for pharmacists to deliver patient targeted services. From a public health view, pharmacists are also involved in health promotion campaigns like tobacco control; moderate alcohol use; nutrition and healthy lifestyle; routine immunization; management and prevention of infectious diseases such as HIV/AIDS, tuberculosis and diarrhea; and in the management of mental health and other chronic diseases [55]. They need to communicate effectively with patients and other colleagues to deliver the best possible collaboration.

Major barriers for effective pharmacy practice in LMICs include a shortage of qualified pharmacists, the pharmacist's preference for working in urban rather than rural areas, failure in the separation of dispensing practices between doctors' clinics and pharmacies, especially in countries where the pharmacists are not the sole dispenser and doctors are allowed to dispense as well, the weak implementation of pharmacy laws, irrational medicine usage, reliance on untrained health workers for delivery of services, and general poverty.

5.2.1. Poor Interprofessional Collaboration

Successful communication between health professionals is a requirement for collaborative practice. Communication and collaboration between pharmacists and other health professions are often asynchronous in different environments and limited to brief interventions related to an individual patient's care. In most practice settings, the focus is on improving medication use, establishing and communicating pharmaceutical care plans, and rectifying prescription or administration errors as well as providing drug information on request [20].

Multiple barriers to effective collaboration between pharmacists and physicians have been identified. External barriers are mostly related to funding and models of care, whereas internal barriers relate to attitudes, beliefs, and the understanding of respective roles. Internal barriers seem to disappear once pharmacists and physicians actually experience collaborative practice and establish a professional relationship. It would be ideal if patients of different kinds of clinicians have a sense of unity in making decision on clinical treatments. Nevertheless, it is only possible when physicians have a high positive attitude of clinical pharmacists and their real contributions [22, 53, 56].

There was also a distinction between pharmacists who already had experience working with other health professionals and health professional students or new graduates. During the reflective process, some realized their preconceived ideas and beliefs about doctors and about how education and training may have influenced their current encounters and past relationships negatively. Some stereotypes of doctors were described as professionally distant and superior who attributed little value to the pharmacist's contributions to team-based healthcare, unless related to rectifying their prescription errors.

Community pharmacists' challenges are to develop a practice-based network that is able to support them and optimize their contribution. Most pharmacists are not affiliated with an institution, and most are often the only pharmacist practising. This indicates the need of providing them with the support of a network of colleagues. If the network connection is not available, some drug-related problems such as adverse effects may regularly occur in patients without the control of pharmacists.

5.2.2. Poor Awareness from Patients

Despite the many approaches listed above, pharmacists are underutilised for patient care in LMICs; and the importance of their role as healthcare professionals in hospitals, community pharmacies and healthcare team have not been well recognized [21, 52, 56]. Pharmacists can be the first point of contact and make appropriate referrals for patients, but patients are sometimes concerned that the pharmacy is running as a business [20].

Adherence and self-management of patients are the conditional factors for good medical practice, especially in patients with chronic illness. They allow patients to take an active part in the management of their own condition [57]. In fact, medical staff often cannot see the patients for months until they come back for follow-up. If patient self-management is not carried out, it causes difficulties in managing the patient illness. Sometimes patients do not tell the whole story for example if they forget to take a dose or used new products that may interfere with their medication. They also may not appreciate follow-ups with pharmacists because they are unfamiliar with the pharmacy profession, they have a perception of insufficient training in disease management, or they simply lack trust [20].

Many patients show their displeasure with the services provided by a pharmacist. They do not trust pharmacist's advice and do not follow the recommendation as they would for a physician's. Some patients believe that pharmacists can be part of the team, but they don't think pharmacists can play a leading role.

5.2.3. Shortage of Investment

Shortage of investment into the public healthcare system is the biggest difficulty for LMICs. For example, the community pharmacist's financial situation worsened, and retirement fund input become lower in recent years in Lebanon. This leads to a lack of employees in the primary healthcare system, and a dependence on untrained employees. Shortages of drugs and equipment are common in public hospitals [58].

In India, a focus on profits, which is the characteristic of certain dispensing practices, rather than the provision of optimal health care promotes irrational use and prescribing of drugs; this issue may not be unique to LMICs. The slowly increasing income of a pharmacist (either owner or employee) is leading to a decrease in the input of pharmacist's retirement pension. Moreover, due to the fierce competition among community pharmacies or private pharmacies, it is difficult to obtain pharmacist assistants (due to worsening financial situation) and many organizations cut down the number of employees, leading to exhaustion and stress in pharmacists due to long working hours [59].

The deteriorating financial situation of the pharmacist seems to be affecting the professionalism of the pharmacist image. In LMICs in Africa, a pharmacist/population ratio of less than 1/100,000 is not uncommon [60]. A similar shortage of pharmacists also occurs in other LMICs.

Developing facilities to enhance the implementation the pharmacist-led approach should also be considered, such as allowing pharmacists to access electronic health records, as well as deregulation of more prescription-only medicines to pharmacy-only medicines.

5.2.4. Problems of Using Incorrect Medicine in Public Health

Antibiotic resistance is alarming in many LMICs due to overusage as well as undertherapeutic-dosage usage. In these communities it is not as easy to make antibiotics charts, assess drug resistance in rural areas and there is loose management of antibiotic use. This causes a serious and widespread public health problem. WHO wishes to amplify the impact of pharmacist interventions and the standard preparation and dispensing in LMICs [61].

The marketing strategy of pharmaceutical companies to boost sales in combination with the desire for modern drugs for preventing diseases are also causes of inappropriate drug use. In addition, cultural norms such as the prevalence of polypharmacy, including combining traditional medicines with allopathic medicines, contribute to the irrational use of drugs [62].

Although the World Health Organization (WHO) is trying to promote Good Pharmacy Practice (GPP) all around the world, pharmacy practice in LMICs is still poor when compared to that in high-income countries. The quality of practice has, however, repeatedly been reported as being low. For example, in India, prescription-only drugs are often sold without a proper diagnosis having been made and prescription given and there is usually a low number of staff in the drugstore, who are not fully qualified. Despite the formal requirements of having a pharmacist present in licensed pharmacies, the pharmacist is recurrently absent [60].

5.3. Ways to Improve the Role of Pharmacists in the Current Healthcare System

Overlapping issues need to be addressed with multiple options. To find proper answers to all, it needs coordination from a proper governance perspective, jointly with all the stakeholders such as the Ministry of Public Health, the Ministry of Education and Higher Education, the universities, and other professional associations. The proposed solutions include the application of good governance principles, provision of Health Insurance services, developing pharmacists' quality and quantity, and new laws and decrees concerning clinical pharmacy application in hospitals and community settings, continuing education consolidation and professional development, and research- and assessment-based decisions. These solutions are expected to overcome challenges and barriers while leveraging careers and promoting it to international standards.

5.3.1. Enhanced Methods of Training

Interprofessional education (IPE) is regarded as a strategy to increase collaboration between health professionals (World Health Organization, 2010). Pharmaceutical accreditation and regulatory agencies and other professional medical university programs recommend and certify IPE as a preparation for professional patient care. Most pharmacy undergraduate programs in Australia offer limited opportunities for IPE and the practice and development of effective interprofessional communication (IPC) skills during undergraduate and/or intern training to enhance clinical pharmacists' confidence in establishing professional relationships, addressing any gaps in their previous training and experience. This prepares them for a more global role as change agents in the quality usage of medicines and medication safety [63, 64]. However, in LMICs, this curriculum has not yet been officially updated, instead, there are short communication skills training courses for medical staff, and policies have been set up in hospitals about communication and collaboration. Changes that occurred in the role of pharmacists on international levels have not been adopted by pharmacists practicing in a traditional way, particularly in the community, when they are available to counsel and provide services. Recently, the concept of medication therapy management (MTM) has been used to describe collaborative methods, with a purpose of achieving optimal patient outcomes and promote safe and effective medication use. MTM services are focused on patient-centered care rather than product-centered care and are targeted to prevent medication-related morbidity and mortality. They can be considered as an activity when pharmacists (including but not limited to hospital and community pharmacists) are reimbursed for reviewing patients' medications and advising them and their careers about necessary changes but without dispensing. MTM services include an assessment of dosing regimen, provision of individual drug records, development of drug-related action plans (which may include therapeutic recommendations and provide referrals), and documentation and follow-up as needed. For patients who are eligible for an MTM program it helps them, and medical staff make sure that their medications are working to improve their health. In addition to simple patient education, MTM consisting of medication optimisation, monitoring of disease control, adverse drug reactions, identification of drug-drug interactions and compliance assessment should also be adopted. Patients can share their ideas and feelings about the illness, moreover, they can share their action plan and medication list [64].

5.3.2. Improving Awareness of Community and Other Healthcare Professionals

Increasing the patient's knowledge and their education on the benefits of adherence to their health and future is essential. It is also advantageous in enhancing the patient's access to the appropriate medications and its safe use

[42]. In modern times, patients are more open and sharing, in addition, patients can find drug information at home by themselves via the internet and newspapers. In patients who have difficulty adhering to treatment such as the elderly patients and patients with comorbidities that need to use a variety of drugs, there are measures such as pill dispensers and reminders, medication schedules and medication reminders via smart electronic devices [62]. Pharmacists should also counsel patients' family members, in order to remind the patients and provide the patients the best caring conditions. In Chile, Thailand, Bulgaria, India, Sudan, Egypt and Paraguay when pharmacists give education and counselling to patients with chronic illnesses: patients experience small improvements in quality of life and patients may use the health services less (for instance fewer visits to the doctor, fewer stays in hospital) [54]. The communication methods for patients and their family members is very important, it must be brief and accurate to help them understand the disease as well as how to use the medicine. To ensure better implementation, the community pharmacy should courage pharmacists to join short-term courses for communication.

Communicating with other healthcare colleagues and building an information network from the community to the hospital has been going well. Although most doctors have no previous experience of cooperative relationships with community pharmacists, most welcomed the concept and highlight the need for increasing awareness of such cooperation. They think this will help reduce the workload for doctors (especially in busy public organizations) and other experts such as nutritionists and physiotherapists who have previously been incorporated in collaborative groups. Other medical staff consider that collaboration will lead to "high-quality work" and "patient-focused teamwork", ensuring appropriate therapy, thanks to the pharmacist for additional safety checks. Moreover, pharmacists' conversation with patients about medications and side effects leads to an increase in their adherence in most cases [54].

To ensure patient privacy and security and the need for continuity and efficiency in communication between pharmacists and physicians, participants suggested that cooperation should be made either based on team group. Focus group discussion depends on the interaction between participants to create data preferred by many researchers because they are an effective way to collect data from a group of participants, and that group interaction allows participants to feel less threatened than in one-on-one interviews, and so participants are able to express their thoughts more freely. Doctors point out the benefits such as reducing drug waste and unnecessary treatments can lead to cost containment in drug budgets in the public organization. The pharmacists were able to learn from the experts within their team; through observation, discussion of problems and expert assessment and feedback [54].

5.3.3. Increasing Quality of Education

Quality of education and training is a priority of the governments. Many medical universities have been established and increasingly improve the quality of teaching [44].

A survey of 89 countries and territories indicated that there were 6 pharmacists per 10,000 population ($n = 80$) but that there is considerable variation between them ranging from 0.02 (Somalia) to 25.07 (Malta) pharmacists per 10,000 population. African nations have significantly fewer pharmacists per capita. Differences emerge with the Africa region which has more pharmacies than pharmacists per capita. Additionally, some countries report more pharmacies than pharmacists (Afghanistan, Bangladesh, Bhutan, Burundi, India, Nepal, Pakistan, Somalia, Vietnam) [65].

Graduate pharmacist numbers from university in the previous years show that the mean ratio of pharmacists is increasing to the global mean.

The oversupply of graduates by universities is increasing, it causes competition between the pharmacists, decreasing the demand (and thus the salary for employed pharmacists), and consequently, it may increase the quality of services offered to patients. The governments and the universities have developed some strategies to curb the exponential increase of pharmacy graduates to maintain the profession; In parallel, there is an adjustment in graduate pharmacist records with international competencies for better jobs being developed, by partnering with academic institutions and relevant authorities. The globalization trend also leads pharmacists to meet international standards, so they are able to work in multinational organizations. In addition, laws need to be updated to conform to international standards and promote change at the practical level. It also enforces the laws, defends the rights of pharmacists, the higher standards improve the level of practice and development of scientific competence.

Emphasising training of public health pharmacists should also be prioritised in developing countries where the need of primary care is unmet. To ensure all graduate pharmacists are prepared to participate in public health activities, education in this field must be provided during their main years of pharmacy school. In the United States and other developed countries, the profession has been trained in secondary preventive care by providing medication to slow the progress of the disease. The ACPE accredits practice-based activities (formerly called Certificate Programs in Pharmacy), which are continuing pharmacy education programs intended to enhance practice through the experiences of advanced knowledge, skills, attitudes, and behaviors [43]. However, in LMICs, the accessibility of pharmacists in preventive health care has presented barriers in applying these methods, but it is still a good start for disease prevention. Prevention focuses on how pharmacists can improve public health, stating the pharmacist's ability to provide prevention medical services related to immunization, cardiovascular risk clinic reduction, smoking cessation clinic and other diseases. Continuing education is a basic step in developing the pharmacist and should not be overlooked. However, unless such training becomes mandatory, there is only small part of the pharmacist community that would engage in it.

Conclusion

Over the years, pharmacy services witnessed a transition of roles of professional practice at the international level. Pharmacists are increasingly being considered an important part of the health care system whether in community pharmacies, primary health centers or hospitals. However, the roles of pharmacists have not been appreciated by patients and other healthcare professionals. Major barriers for effective pharmacy practice in

LMICs include a shortage of qualified pharmacists, the pharmacist's preference of working area, failure in communication between doctors and pharmacists, the weak implementation of pharmacy laws, a reliance on untrained health workers for delivery of services, and general poverty.

Although many difficulties still exist, pharmaceutical practice is getting more and more attention from the community and the governments. Strategies and laws have been designed to guarantee the rights and obligations of pharmacists. Education is increasingly being improved to strengthen the quality of graduated pharmacists. It has to be developed gradually with the support of government and the renovation of healthcare service delivery, including developing facilitating measures to extend pharmacists' responsibilities.

REFERENCES

[1] World Health Organization. The pharmacist in the health care system: report of a WHO consultative group, New Delhi, India, 13-16 December 1988; *report of a WHO meeting*, Tokyo, Japan, 31 August - 3 September 1993.

[2] Bender, GA; Thom, RA. *Great Moments in Pharmacy*. Northwood Institute Press.

[3] Bigoniya, P. *Adverse Drug Reaction Reporting: The Essential Component of Pharmacovigilance*.

[4] Carter, BL. Evolution of Clinical Pharmacy in the US and Future Directions for Patient Care. *Drugs Aging*. 2016 Mar, 33(3), 169-77.

[5] Bhagavathula, AS; Sarkar, BR; Patel, I. Clinical pharmacy practice in developing countries: Focus on India and Pakistan. *Archives of Pharmacy Practice*., V. 5, I. 2, April-Jun 2014, 91-94.

[6] Saseen, JJ; Ripley, TL; Bondi, D; et al. ACCP Clinical Pharmacist Competencies. *Pharmacotherapy*., 2017 May, 37(5), 630-636.

[7] Morak, S; Vogler, S; Walser, et al. Vienna: Austrian Federal Ministry of Health; 2010. *Understanding the pharmaceutical care concept and applying it in practice*.

[8] Ashenef, A. Assessment of the Use and Status of New Drug Information Centers in a Developing Country, Ethiopia: The Case of Public University Hospital Drug Information Centers. *BioMed Research International*, 2018, (3), 1-11.

[9] Vidotti, CCF. Drug information Centers in developing countries and the promotion of rational use of drugs: A viewpoint about challenges and perspectives. *Int. Pharm. J.*, V. 18, N. 1, 2004, 21-23.

[10] Fornasier, G; Taborelli, M; Francescon, S. Targeted therapies and adverse drug reactions in oncology: the role of clinical pharmacist in pharmacovigilance. *Int J Clin Pharm.*, 2018 Aug, 40(4), 795-802.

[11] Shamim, S; Sharib, SM; Malhi, SM. *Adverse drug reactions (ADRS) reporting: awareness and reasons of under-reporting among health care professionals, a challenge for pharmacists.* Springerplus., 2016, Oct 12, 5(1), 1778.

[12] Manias, E. Effects of interdisciplinary collaboration in hospitals on medication errors: an integrative review. *Expert Opin Drug Saf.*, 2018 Mar, 17(3), 259-275.

[13] Guchelaar, H; Colen, HBB; Kalmeijer, MD. Medication Errors Hospital Pharmacist Perspective. *Drugs.*, 2005, 65(13), 1735-46.

[14] Mekonnen, AB; McLachlan, AJ; Brien, JE. Evaluation of the impact of pharmacist-led medication reconciliation intervention: a single centre pre–post study from Ethiopia. *Int J Clin Pharm.*, 2018, Oct, 40(5), 1209-1216.

[15] Chalasani, SH; Ramesh, M; Gurumurthy, P. Pharmacist-Initiated Medication Error-Reporting and Monitoring Programme in a Developing Country Scenario. *Pharmacy* (Basel)., 2018 Dec, 6(4), 133.

[16] Huong-Thao Nguyen, Hong-Tham Pham, Dang-Khoa Vo. The effect of a clinical pharmacistled training programme on intravenous medication errors: a controlled before and after study. *BMJ Qual Saf.*, 2014 Apr, 23(4), 319-24.

[17] Rekha, M; Mubeena, T. A study on role of Clinical Pharmacist in identification and reporting of drug interactions in Physciatric Ward in

a Teritary Care Teaching Hospital. *Indian journal of pharmacy practice*, 11(4), 198-203.

[18] Martin, P; Tamblyn, R; Benedetti, A. Effect of a Pharmacist-Led Educational Intervention on Inappropriate Medication Prescriptions in Older Adults. The D-PRESCRIBE Randomized Clinical Trial. *JAMA.*, 2018 Nov, 13, 320(18), 1889-1898.

[19] E-Silveira, D; EM-Villalba, F; Freire, MG. The impact of Pharmacy Intervention on the treatment of elderly multi-pathological patients. *Farm Hosp.*, 2015, Jul 1, 39(4), 192-202.

[20] Wong, FY; Chan, FW; You, JH. Patient self-management and pharmacist-led patient self-management in Hong Kong: A focus group study from different healthcare professionals' perspectives. *BMC Health Serv Res.*, 2011 May, 24, 11, 121.

[21] McCullough, MB; Petrakis, B; Christopher Gillespie, MPA. Knowing the patient: A qualitative study on care-taking and the clinical pharmacist-patient relationship. *Research in Social and Administrative Pharmacy.*, 2016 Jan-Feb, 12(1), 78-90.

[22] Ismail, S; Osman, M; Abulezz, R. Pharmacists as Interprofessional Collaborators and Leaders through Clinical Pathway. *Pharmacy (Basel).*, 2018 Mar, 16, 6(1), pii: E24.

[23] Guénette, L; Maheu, A; Vanier, M. Pharmacists practising in family medicine groups: What are their activities and needs? *Journal of Clinical Pharmacy and Therapeutics.*, August 2019.

[24] Gerber, BS; Rapacki, L; Castillo, A. Design of a trial to evaluate the impact of clinical pharmacists and community health promoters working with African-Americans and Latinos with Diabetes. *BMC Public Health.*, 2012, Oct 23, 12, 891.

[25] Sharp, LK; Tilton, JJ; Touchette, DR. Community Health Workers Supporting Clinical Pharmacists in Diabetes Management: A Randomized-Controlled Trial. *Pharmacotherapy.*, 2018 Jan, 38(1), 58-68.

[26] Jeong, S; Lee, M; Ji, E. Effect of pharmaceutical care interventions on glycemic control in patients with diabetes: a systematic review and meta-analysis. *Ther Clin Risk Manag.*, 2018, Sep 28, 14, 1813-1829.

[27] Marfo, A; Owusu, F-Daaku. Exploring the extended role of the community pharmacist in improving blood pressure control among hypertensive patients in a developing setting. *J Pharm Policy Pract.*, 2017, Dec 21, 10, 39.

[28] Jahangard, Z.-Rafsanjani, Sarayani, A; Nosrati, M. Effect of a Community Pharmacist–Delivered Diabetes Support Program for Patients Receiving Specialty Medical Care. A Randomized Controlled Trial. *Diabetes Educ.*, 2015 Feb, 41(1), 127-35.

[29] Smitha, MT; Monahana, MP; Nelson, P. Elevated blood pressure in the developing world: a role for clinical pharmacists. *Int J Pharm Pract.*, 2018 Aug, 26(4), 334-340.

[30] Schwalm, JD; McKee, M; Huffman, MD; et al. *Resource Effective Strategies to Prevent and Treat Cardiovascular Disease. Circulation.*, 2016, Feb 23, 133(8), 742–755.

[31] Upadhyay, D; Ibrahim, M; Mishra, P. Does pharmacist-supervised intervention through pharmaceutical care program influence direct healthcare cost burden of newly diagnosed diabetics in a tertiary care teaching hospital in Nepal: a non-clinical randomised controlled trial approach. *Daru.*, 2016, Feb 29, 24, 6.

[32] Polgreen, LA. Cost effectiveness of a physician-pharmacist collaboration intervention to improve blood pressure control. *Hypertension.*, 2015 Dec, 66(6), 1145-51.

[33] Chen, J; Lu, XY; Wang, WJ; et al. Cheng B Impact of a Clinical Pharmacist-Led Guidance Team on Cancer Pain Therapy in China: A Prospective Multicenter Cohort Study. *J Pain Symptom Manage.*, 2014 Oct, 48(4), 500-9.

[34] Zhang, Y; Wang, Y; Xiao, Z. Pharmacists' roles in cancer pain control: A model in developing China. *Res Social Adm Pharm.*, 2015, May-Jun, 11(3), e144-5.

[35] Sharma, S; Khanal, T; Shrestha, S. A celebration of World Pharmacist Day 2018 focusing to strengthen the pharmacy services at an oncology-based hospital in Nepal: Inspiration for others in developing countries. *Res Social Adm Pharm.*, 2019 Jan, 15(1), 117-118.

[36] Sakeenal, MHF; Bennett, AA; McLachlan, AJ. Enhancing pharmacists' role in developing countries to overcome the challenge of antimicrobial resistance: a narrative review. *Antimicrob Resist Infect Control.*, 2018, May 2, 7, 63.

[37] Haque, A; Hussain, K; Ibrahim, R. Impact of pharmacist-led antibiotic stewardship program in a PICU of low/middle-income country. *BMJ Open Qual.*, 2018, Jan 6, 7(1), e000180.

[38] Saengcharoen, W; Jaisawang, P; Udomcharoensab, P; et al. Appropriateness of diagnosis of streptococcal pharyngitis among Thai community pharmacists according to the Centor criteria. *Int J Clin Pharm.*, 2016 Oct, 38(5), 1318-25.

[39] WHO. *The role of pharmacist in encouraging prudent use of antibiotics and averting antimicrobial resistance: a review of policy and experience.*

[40] Tängdén, T; Ramos Martín, V; Felton, TW. *The role of infection models and PK/PD modelling for optimising care of critically ill patients with severe infections.*, (2017).

[41] Mossialos, E; Courtin, E; Naci, H; Benrimoj, S; Bouvy, M; Farris, K; Sketris, I. From "retailers" to health care providers: Transforming the role of community pharmacists in chronic disease management. *Health Policy*, (2015), 119(5), 628–639.

[42] Barry, AR; Pammett, RT. Applying the guidelines for pharmacists integrating into primary care teams. *Canadian Pharmacists Journal / Revue Des Pharmaciens Du Canada*, (2016), 149(4), 219–225.

[43] American College of Clinical Pharmacy. Desired professional development pathways for clinical pharmacists. *Pharmacotherapy.*, 2013 Apr, 33(4), e34-42.

[44] Murad, MS; Chatterley, T; Guirguis, LM. A meta-narrative review of recorded patient–pharmacist interactions: Exploring biomedical or patient-centered communication? *Research in Social and Administrative Pharmacy*, (2014), 10(1), 1–20.

[45] Murad, MS; Chatterley, T; Guirguis, LM. A meta-narrative review of recorded patient–pharmacist interactions: Exploring biomedical or

patient-centered communication? *Research in Social and Administrative Pharmacy*, (2014), 10(1), 1–20.

[46] Hindi, AMK; Schafheutle, EI; Jacobs, S. Community pharmacy integration within the primary care pathway for people with long-term conditions: a focus group study of patients', pharmacists' and GPs' experiences and expectations. *BMC Family Practice*, (2019), 20(1).

[47] Donald, M; King-Shier, K; Tsuyuki, RT; Al Hamarneh, YN; Jones, CA; Manns, B; Hemmelgarn, BR. Patient, family physician and community pharmacist perspectives on expanded pharmacy scope of practice: a qualitative study. *CMAJ Open*, (2017), 5(1), E205–E212.

[48] Khanal, S; Nissen, L; Veerman, L; Hollingworth, S. Pharmacy workforce to prevent and manage non-communicable diseases in developing nations: The case of Nepal. *Research in Social and Administrative Pharmacy*, (2016), 12(4), 655–659.

[49] Gray, NJ; Shaw, KL; Smith, FJ; Burton, J; Prescott, J; Roberts, R; McDonagh, JE. The Role of Pharmacists in Caring for Young People with Chronic Illness. *Journal of Adolescent Health*, (2017), 60(2), 219–225.

[50] Gray, NJ; Shaw, KL; Smith, FJ; Burton, J; Prescott, J; Roberts, R; McDonagh, JE. The Role of Pharmacists in Caring for Young People with Chronic Illness. *Journal of Adolescent Health*, (2017), 60(2), 219–225.

[51] Wahab, MSA. The relevance of educating doctors, pharmacists and older patients about potentially inappropriate medications. *International Journal of Clinical Pharmacy*, (2015), 37(6), 971–974.

[52] Wahab, MSA. The relevance of educating doctors, pharmacists and older patients about potentially inappropriate medications. *International Journal of Clinical Pharmacy*, (2015), 37(6), 971–974.

[53] Christin Löffler1 *, et al*. Perceptions of interprofessional collaboration of general practitioners and community pharmacists - a qualitative study. *BMC Health Services Research.*, (2017).

[54] Pande, S; Hiller, JE; Nkansah, N; Bero, L. The effect of pharmacist-provided non-dispensing services on patient outcomes, health service

utilisation and costs in low- and middle-income countries. *Cochrane Database of Systematic Reviews.*, (2013).

[55] Law, MG; Maposa, P; Steeb, DR; Duncan, G. Addressing the global need for public health clinical pharmacists through student pharmacist education: a focus on developing nations. *International Journal of Clinical Pharmacy*, (2017), 39(6), 1141–1144.

[56] Reeves, S; Pelone, F; Harrison, R; Goldman, J; Zwarenstein, M. Interprofessional collaboration to improve professional practice and healthcare outcomes. *Cochrane Database of Systematic Reviews.*, (2017).

[57] Foster, G; Taylor, SJC; Eldridge, S; Ramsay, J; Griffiths, CJ. Self-management education programmes by lay leaders for people with chronic conditions. *Cochrane Database of Systematic Reviews*, 2007, 4, CD005108.

[58] Hala Sacre, Souheil Hallit, Aline Hajj, Rony M Zeenny, Georges Sili, Pascale Salameh. The pharmacy profession in a developing country: Challenges and suggested governance solutions in Lebanon. *J Res Pharm Pract.*, 2019 Apr-Jun, 8(2), 39-44.

[59] Sabde, YD; Diwan, V; Saraf, VS; Mahadik, VK; Diwan, VK; De Costa, A. Mapping private pharmacies and their characteristics in Ujjain district, Central India. *BMC Health Services Research*, (2011), 11(1). *BMC Health Services Research*, volume 11.

[60] Sabde, YD; Diwan, V; Saraf, VS; Mahadik, VK; Diwan, VK; De Costa, A. Mapping private pharmacies and their characteristics in Ujjain district, Central India. BMC Health Services Research, (2011), 11(1). *BMC Health Services Research*, volume 11.

[61] Dalton, K; Byrne, S. Role of the pharmacist in reducing healthcare costs: current insights. *Integrated Pharmacy Research and Practice*, (2017), Volume 6, 37–46.

In: Pharmacists
Editor: Line L. Villadsen

ISBN: 978-1-53618-018-3
© 2020 Nova Science Publishers, Inc.

Chapter 5

SYNTHESIS OF RELEVANT INFORMATION TO SUPPORT MULTI-CRITERIA DECISION ANALYSIS (MCDA) FOR PHARMACIST DECISION-MAKING

Alberto Frutos Pérez-Surio[*]

Pharmacy Department, University Lozano Blesa Clinical Hospital, Zaragoza, Spain
Microbiology, Preventive Medicine and Public Health Department, University of Zaragoza, Zaragoza, Spain

ABSTRACT

Introduction: Decision-making in healthcare is often complex and involves consideration of numerous factors, hence many of these processes require careful assessment of existing health technologies, as well as the consideration of multiple dimensions to analyze the value of available options.

---

[*] Corresponding Author's Email: ajfrutos@unizar.es; ajfrutos@salud.aragon.es

Currently, some countries support macro and meso decision-making in the field of health on economic concepts, with the budgetary impact of the technologies being a major criterion. Further, the Anglo-Saxon model based on cost-utility analysis is used, which provides an estimate that relates the Quality Adjusted Life Years (QALYs) with the costs of health technology. Such analysis is widely used by health technology assessment (HTA) agencies, academia, as well as in industry.

However, value and its dimensions are more complex if we seek to make decisions based on the value of medications. The use of structured and explicit approaches that require the evaluation of multiple criteria containing value dimensions can significantly improve the quality of pharmacy decision-making. Multi-criteria decision analysis (MCDA) is a complementary decision-making tool that can systematically incorporate, in addition to the costs and benefits of medical innovations, other dimensions such as ethical, organisational, legal, environmental and social aspects, together with the perspectives of the various stakeholders.

Aims and Objectives: The objective of this review is to make a proposal for the implementation of the analysis of ethical, organisational, legal, social, environmental and other domains, in the studies of the HTA agencies, enabling the incorporation of well-informed MCDA approaches into pharmacist decision-making.

Methods:

- In order to know the scientific evidence on MCDA techniques in which non-core criteria were used or included for decision-making on the incorporation, modification or exclusion of health technologies, a systematic review was carried out using structured searches in biomedical databases and webpages of different HTA organisations, to sum up the criteria that should be part of each of the aforementioned non-core domains.

Results:

- As a result of the search for scientific evidence, 42 articles were included that used non-core criteria for the evaluation of health technologies. A total of 216 non-core criteria were extracted and classified by the researchers from these articles, of which 56 were included in the social (socioeconomic) domain, 59 in the organizational, 10 in the legal, 8 in the environmental, 47 in the ethical and 36 in other domains.
- Of the 216 non-core criteria obtained from the systematic review, 26 criteria were necessary for pharmacist decision-making. These criteria were grouped by domain as follows: five criteria for each of the

ethical, legal and environmental domains, four for the social domain and the other domain, and three for the organizational domain.

Conclusion:

- The 26 selected criteria should be considered by HTA agencies when collecting and synthesizing information for pharmacist decision-making.
- The consensus group does not consider that some of the domains should be weighed above others or that some individual criteria are more preeminent than others.
- It is proposed to use MCDA models within a deliberative process and to include it in the information to be retrieved in the process of evaluation of health technologies.
- These models can serve as a frame of reference in a systematic and structured discussion based on individual criteria and the evidence supporting them.
- Structured and informed deliberative models have a certain advantage over closed and uninformed decision-making processes, as they make explicit and transparent the reasoning behind the final decision.

Keywords: pharmacist, multicriteria decision analysis, health technology assessment

INTRODUCTION

Pharmacist decision-making is often complex and multifaceted. Many of these decisions require a careful evaluation of existing health technologies and their position within the management pathway in a particular context (e.g., pharmacotherapy, etc.), as well as the use of multiple criteria to evaluate available alternatives.

Currently, some countries base macro- and meso- decision-making on fundamentally economic concepts for coverage, reimbursement and pricing (budgetary impact and cost-effectiveness). The arguments behind these concepts are based on a comparison of the costs and benefits of different health services (health technology), understood as pharmaceuticals, medical devices, public health interventions, organisational models or surgical procedures. Few countries take into account the fourth guarantee (economic analysis) for decision-making. In fact, it is only used when the assessment of incremental effectiveness and safety (defined differently by countries) does not allow consensus to be reached in regulatory/industry negotiations, as, for example, in Germany (Campillo-Artero C et al., 2018; Culyer AJ, 2014; Campillo-Artero C and Puig-Junoy J, 2018). In most cases this comparison is made using the Anglo-Saxon model based on cost-benefit analysis, which provides an estimate of Quality Adjusted Life Years (QALYs) relative to the costs of healthcare technology. This analysis is widely used by health technology assessment (HTA) agencies, academia and industry because QALYs are assumed to be an objective measure for comparing health technologies, even if they do not always support the decision as the sole criterion in all settings.

This is a method used in some countries (mainly English-speaking) attractive for the determination of a numerical result and the possibility of comparing technologies for the same pathology or condition and/or between pathologies, in making decisions on the incorporation, diffusion or exclusion of health technologies. But apart from the health costs and benefits of these, there are many other aspects/dimensions that have to be taken into account such as: degree of innovation of the new technology, acceptability, accessibility and ethical, organizational, legal, environmental, social, etc. aspects. It should also include perspectives of each of the parties involved in the implementation or exclusion of health technologies (patients, payers, etc.), since for each of them health technology can have a different benefit and the important results can be different.

The use of structured and explicit approaches that require multi-criteria assessment can significantly improve the quality of pharmacist decision-making. A complementary decision-making tool that can systematically incorporate, in addition to the costs and benefits of medical innovations, other dimensions such as ethical, organisational, legal and social aspects, along with the perspectives of different stakeholders, is Multicriteria Decision Analysis (MCDA).

The main aspects of any MCDA method are: 1) the alternatives to be evaluated; 2) the criteria (or attributes) against which the alternatives are evaluated; 3) the scores of the criteria that reflect the value of the expected performance of each of the alternatives; and 4) weights of criteria that measure the relative importance of each criterion in comparison with others. MCDA approaches, in general, can be classified into three categories: value measurement models, exceedance approach, and mode- target, aspiration, or reference level models (Thokala P et al., 2012).

Given the diversity of MCDA methods (Marsh et al., 2014), the user is faced with the challenge not only of how to put it into practice, but also in what terms of the fundamental theories and knowledge on which they are based. The current literature on health MCDA offers little guidance on: 1) how to choose from the overwhelming variety of approaches; 2) which is the "best" approach for different types of decisions; and 3) what are the relevant considerations. The lack of guidance on how to implement MCDA techniques in health can cause the MCDA to be misused and decision-makers to be misled (Mullen, 2004) by the incorporation of models that do not take into account all the dimensions or at least those that are accepted or assumed in that environment as important and in the weight that is to be given, always based on the context of application and its characteristics.

In order to address this lack of guidance, the International Society for Pharmacoeconomics and Outcomes Research (ISPOR) established an Emerging Good Practice Working Group to determine a definition for the MCDA and to develop a good practice guide for the conduct of MCDA to contribute to pharmacist decision-making. Two reports were made during 2016. In the first report, the MCDA was defined.

In addition, it was suggested that it would be useful to consider the types of pharmacist decision-making, describing the key steps involved, and finally providing an overview of MCDA's main methods (Thokala P et al., 2016). In the second report, a good practice guide was provided that included how to select the "right" MCDA job for each type of decision and how to implement their approaches. A checklist was also available for those conducting an MCDA (Marsh K et al., 2016).

The advantages that these models can bring to decision-making seem certain, as they cover all the domains that provide evidence and influence whether decisions are accepted, can be explicitly prioritised and respond to the maximum of public basin surrender. However, for such models to work they must receive evidence inputs from all domains to be considered, otherwise they will be partial and biased.

To date, work has been carried out by international networks such as European Network for Health Technology Assessment (EUnetHTA) or International Network of Agencies for Health Technology Assessment (INAHTA) on the homogenisation of the so-called "core" analyses, including economic evaluation. However, although there are structural models for addressing the problem, such as the EVIDEM (Evidence and Value: Impact on DEcisionMaking) developed by the non-profit organisation EVIDEM Collaboration, the Local HTA Decision-Support Program developed by the University of Calgary or the MEAT (Most Economic Advantageous Tender) framework evaluated by the private organisation MedTech Europe, no other analyses have been standardised that would support areas such as ethical, legal, social, cultural or organisational evaluation. Failure to delve into such analyses would leave any decision-making attempt incomplete. Likewise, new domains have appeared which, although considered in a few environments, may have some importance in the future, such as those relating to the environmental impact of the production, translation, use and recycling or disposal of health technologies.

Given the current trend to include in the decision-making in HTA, in addition to the "core" domains, the so-called "non-core" ones, there is a need to produce a report analysing the current level of development and depth of the so-called "non-core" domains (other than clinical and economic) in the pharmacist decision-making process for incorporation, modification or exclusion of health technologies (ethical, legal, organisational, environmental, social and other aspects) by national and international HTA agencies and the models that have been developed in other environments to make these analyses visible and facilitate them. In addition, the assignment included the drafting of a proposal for the implementation of "non-core" domain analyses in agency reports and therefore the information that would enable MCDA decision-making models to be responded to in their different context-dependent formulations.

The general objective was to analyze the current level of development, under MCDA criteria, of the ethical, legal, social, cultural, environmental, organizational or other domains by the national and international HTA agencies that have developed to make such analysis visible and facilitate. The specific objective was to make a proposal for the implementation of "non-core" analyses in the reports of the HTA agencies, which will allow a response to the MCDA decision-making models.

METHODS

Systematic Review of Literature

A systematic review of the evidence was conducted, with no time limit for onset and up to October 2017, consisting of a published literature search on MCDA techniques employing or including 'non-core' criteria for decision-making in the incorporation, modification or exclusion of health technologies. The biomedical databases Medline (PubMed) and Embase were searched.

The specific search strategy designed included, among others, the following terms in free and/or controlled language: Multi Criteria Decision Analysis or MCDA.

The search strategy was adapted to each of the databases following the following structure:

1. (multi-criteria or multicriteria or multiple criteria or multiple-criteria or "multiple criteria" or "multi criteria")
2. "decision*"
3. 1 and 2
4. (mcda or mcdm)
5. 3 or 4
6. (patient* or population) or (social or societ* or communit*) or (ethic* or equit* or equal* or valu*) or (law* or statut* or amendment* or plan* or legal* or legislat* or regulation* or

regulator* or polic* or mandate* or normative*) or (politic* or cultur* or historic* or context* or environment*) or (organization*)
7. 5 and 6
8. (decision and mak*) or (health or healthcare or "health care" or health-care) or (medic* or disease* or pharma*)
9. 7 and 8

Selected databases (Web of Science) and nursing databases (CINAHL) were also searched, as well as pages of different HTA organisations to find out what publications existed on the subject. Similarly, references of included papers were manually reviewed in order to locate studies not retrieved in automated searches.

A search update was performed to identify new studies prior to final editing of the review.

Articles that could be relevant based on their title and abstract were selected by two independent researchers for full text reading based on the following inclusion and exclusion criteria:

- Inclusion criteria: original articles, systematic reviews and procurement guides published in peer-reviewed journals until October 2017 in English or Spanish, which developed MCDA models based on domains or "non-core" criteria to inform HTA decision-making.
- Exclusion criteria: articles, systematic reviews or procurements guides that did not include MCDA models, that did not use these models to inform decisions in the HTA and that although developing MCDA models for this reason, were only based on "core" domains. Documents published on web pages, communiqués to congresses, letters to the editor, editorials and comments, were also excluded.

The selected articles were described in tables designed "ad hoc". These included the author of the article, the domains and criteria analysed, their definition and the healthcare technology evaluated.

The "non-core" criteria extracted from the selected articles were classified and grouped in a table in the following domains: social (socioeconomic), organizational, legal, environmental, ethical and others.

Since the research question addressed is a non-clinical one, no formal evaluation of the methodological quality of the evidence was considered necessary.

RESULTS

Bibliographic Search

Thanks to the bibliographic strategy, 2,859 articles were recovered (Figure 1) of which 1,431 were excluded either because of the type of study or language or because they were duplicated. 1,428 studies were reviewed by title and abstract following the inclusion and exclusion criteria specified in the methodology section. Finally, 42 articles were selected and included for the analysis and summary. In the search update, conducted in May 2018, no articles relevant to the study were identified.

The systematic review showed that MCDA models were used in countries with different economic development and health systems. They were most often used in high-income European countries (Germany, Italy, France, Spain, Poland, Bulgaria, Ireland) or Canada, although in some cases they were used in middle- or low-income countries such as Thailand, Morocco, Iran, Ghana or Colombo.

The MCDA models analyzed in the different articles evaluated a high number of health technologies with different innovation range. They were used to analyze drugs (no patent, orphan or new), public health programs (HIV, obesity), medical devices (cardiac sensors, surgical assistance robots, root screws for lumbar arthrodesis), treatments in general (oncology, Turner syndrome, Lyme disease). Some studies evaluated one or a few interventions, while others analysed up to 56.

In addition, articles were retrieved in which mode- the general MCDA were developed for decision-making in HTA, some of them based on the EVIDEM framework. Four systematic reviews were also retrieved.

Studies were conducted at different levels of decision-making. The majority were carried out at the national level, although there was some which was carried out at the regional level or at the hospitalarian level.

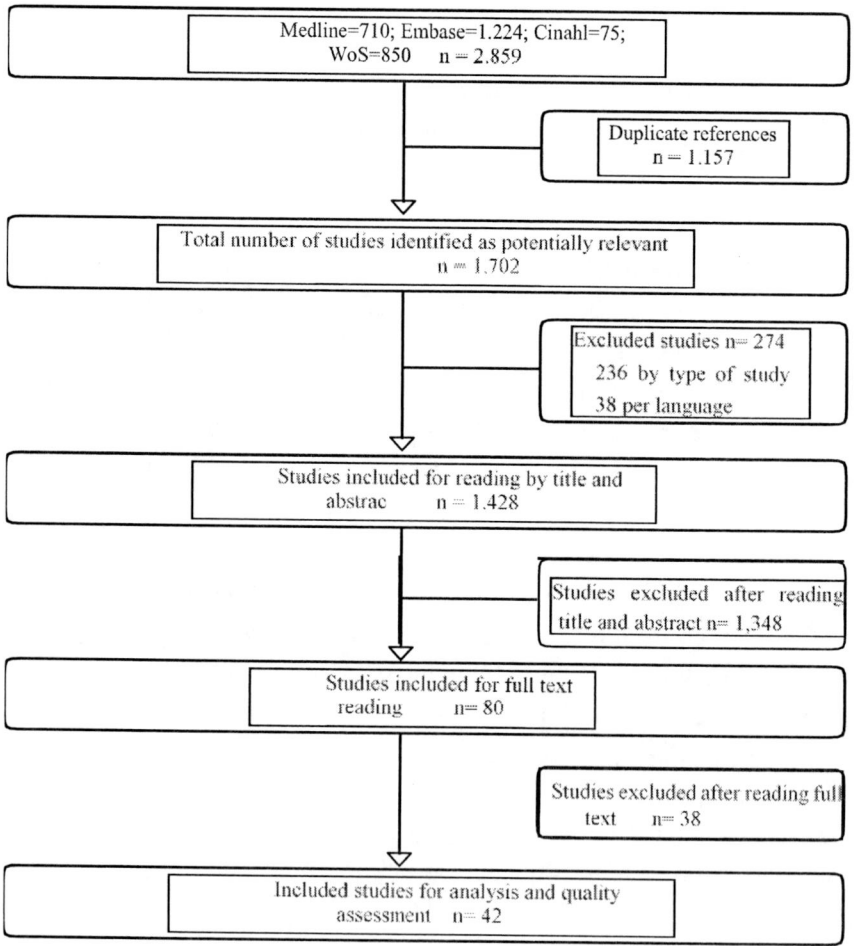

Figure 1. Flowchart.

Of the 42 articles analyzed, the "non-core" criteria were obtained, which were used in them for the HTA. These criteria were grouped into the social (socioeconomic), organizational, legal, environmental, ethical and other domains. A total of 216 criteria were extracted and classified as "non-core" by the researchers, of which: 56 criteria were included in the social (socio-economic) domain, 59 in the organisation, 10 in the legal domain, 8 in the environmental domain, 47 in the ethical domain and 36 in others.

The final product obtained through the consensus group, i.e., the criteria for each domain as well as its definition, are reflected in Tables 1, 2, 3, 4, 5 and 6.

Table 1. Definition criteria Ethical Domain

Criteria-Ethical Domain	Definition
Adequate transmission of information to the patient and/or representative.	Providing health information in a comprehensible and appropriate manner (in time and form) to the patient or his/her representative.
Equity, impartiality, justice and gender mainstreaming.	Everyone, regardless of income, sex, race, age, religion, background, health status or availability of treatment, should have a fair and equal opportunity to live a full healthy life.
Reduction of poverty and inequality.	Guarantee of preferential access to the socio-health system for disadvantaged populations (people with lower incomes have a greater need for support and tend to have a worse state of health) and vulnerable groups (people with mental disorder, disability or functional diversity, victims of abuse or neglect, victims of violence against women, immigrants in irregular administrative situations, excluded personnel or at risk of social exclusion and transsexual persons).
Empowerment of citizens/patients.	Provision of tools for training citizens and patients in joint decision-making.
Ethical conflicts related to the use of technology.	Preservation of privacy/privacy and use of big data; risk/benefit assessment of technology deployment; dehumanization.

Table 2. Definition criteria Legal Domain

Criteria-Legal Domain	Definition
Need for legislative development of norms, directives, accreditations and/or transpositions.	The implantation, adaptation or elimination of the technology could require a normative development that accompanies it.
Need to verify compliance with specific regulations.	The implementation, adaptation or elimination of technology may require the establishment of mechanisms to monitor compliance with regulations and people.
Alignment with plans, protocols, strategic lines.	Adaptation of the use of technology to the existing guidelines in the health system in which it is intended to be implemented.
Verification of compliance with data protection principles/ implementation of specific measures to that effect.	The implementation, adaptation or elimination of technology may require the establishment of measures to ensure confidentiality and the appropriate use of data in accordance with current legislation.
Verification of respect for the patient's autonomy.	The implementation, adaptation or elimination of technology may require ensuring that patient autonomy is respected at all stages of the process, including advance directives.

Table 3. Definition of criteria Organizational Domain

Criteria-Organizational Domain	Definition
Impact of technology and technical, institutional and operational implementation capacity.	Availability of infrastructures, organisation (possibility of integrating technology into the existing health organisation or creating a new one), human resources (quantity, quality and training), skills for the introduction (acceptability) and proper use of health technology (adequacy).
Patient-centered care organization.	The characteristics of the patient could define the actions to be taken on him.
Alignment with context priorities and long-term impact.	Adequacy with the demand and the priorities of the environment that could have an impact on the results of the health system.

Table 4. Definition of Social Domain criteria

Criteria - Social dominance	Definition
Social determinants of health and their impact.	Technology could influence sociodemographic characteristics and their involvement in health.
Socio-economic risks and benefits for the groups affected by the technology, with special attention to the impact on vulnerable groups.	Technology implies a modification of the socioeconomic status of the affected groups, especially in vulnerable groups.
Impact on health prevention.	Technology affects the determinants related to the development of the pathology or condition or to its natural course.
Patient participation and value of their experiences and needs in decision-making.	Ensuring patient participation in decision-making at all levels, including their experiences and preferences.

Table 5. Definition of criteria Domain Environment

Criteria-Domain Environment	Definition
Need to manage waste.	Technology requires the treatment of the waste it generates.
Environmental impact of technology manufacturing.	The production of the technology has an impact on the environment.
Environmental impact of the use of technology.	The use of technology has an impact on the environment.
Scheduled obsolescence and its implications.	The expiry of the planned technology has an added environmental impact.
Environmental impact of the elimination of technology by users.	Once the technology is used, its disposal by users has environmental consequences.

This methodological report attempts to respond to the need to incorporate qualitative criteria, also known as contextual criteria, through systematic and transparent processes in pharmacist decision-making for the introduction, modification and elimination of health technologies. To this end, a proposal has been drawn up for the implementation of "non-core" domain analyses (ethical, legal, social, organisational, environmental and others) in agency reports and therefore provide information that will enable MCDA decision-making models to be responded to in their different context-dependent formulations.

In accordance with the Good Practice Guidance for Conducting MCDA to Contribute to Health Decision Making by an ISPOR Emerging Good Practice Working Group (Marsh K et al., 2016), the corresponding criteria were selected and structured. For this purpose, a systematic search was made of the published literature on MCDA techniques in which "non-core" criteria were used or included for decision-making in the incorporation, modification or exclusion of health technologies and the discussion these criteria in order to select and define those considered most important.

Table 6. Definition of criteria Domain Other

Criteria-Domain Other	Definition
Timeliness and usefulness of health technology assessment.	Whether or not an assessment of health technologies is carried out during their life cycle may lead to a change in the use of such technologies.
Alignment with Profarma plan and contribution to GDP (National).	The health technology is developed by the local, regional, national company and its interaction with the health system results in an improvement in the GDP.
Innovation of the intervention and previous congruence.	The change generated by the technology adapts to the previous application framework.
Technovigilance and cybersecurity.	The need to identify, prevent and resolve events or incidents related to the use of technology through causality assessment and risk management in order to prevent their occurrence and ensure the protection of sensitive information assets.

The decision-making model proposed in this report includes some of the characteristics of the MCDA (criteria, consensus statement) but does not incorporate its mathematical elements (scoring the alternatives, weighting the criteria and calculating an aggregate score). What is proposed is to develop a deliberative process that proposes the de-bat on the selected criteria, thus complying with the broader definition given by ISPOR for MCDA: "methods that aid deliberative discussion using explicitly defined criteria, but without quantitative modelling" (Thokala P et al., 2016).

Why is a deliberative process proposed? As Culyer (Culyer JA, 2014) indicates, a deliberative process is participatory and is often followed by a period of consultation with relevant stakeholders. It involves obtaining and combining various types of evidence in order to arrive at an evidence-based trial. In addition, as Poulin (Poulin P et al., 2013) points out, if individual criteria are not weighted to reflect their importance, the relevance of a particular criterion may change on a case- by-case basis. Therefore, use in the MCDA a deliberative process to make recommendations for HTA is best suited by providing guidance for systematic discussion and a clear understanding of how each criterion and its related evidence impacts on the final discussion. Younkon, Jehu- Appiah and Tanios (Younkong S et al., 2012; Jehu-Appiah C et al., 2008; Tanios N et al, 2013) note that MCDAs should include a deliberative process to address non-quantitative concerns (assessments of ethical and social acceptability as well as the complexity of the intervention) and encourage balanced judgments on intervention priorities in order to reach consensus by stakeholders by facilitating debate and decisions across jurisdictions, decision levels and perspectives (Frutos et al., 2019a; Frutos et al., 2019b; Frutos et al., 2019c; Frutos et al. 2018; Frutos et al. 2016).

In addition, several authors suggest a series of concerns at the time of granting weights and weightings to criteria in MCDA that reaffirms us in the adoption of the proposed deliberative model. Thus Phelps (Phelps CE et al., 2017) indicates that the weight adjustment protocol in the process of analytical hierarchy may allow internal inconsistencies and the re-view of rank or change in the hierarchical order of desirability between different decision options. Marsh (Marsh KD et al., 2017) points out that since weights express trade-offs between degrees of performance on criterion scales, interested parties charged with pro- veering them need to keep scale ranges in mind, so weights should not be tendered regardless of the range of consequences.

Another concern that may arise is how potentially divergent weights of different stakeholders can be accommodated (Younkong S et al., 2012). Given the subjective nature of weights, as they reflect the multifaceted meaning and values determined by stakeholders (Hosikawa K et al., 2016), it is difficult to assess their apparent validity without a precise definition of the criteria (Marsh KD et al., 2017), as they can establish weights in unexpected ways (Hosikawa K et al., 2016) producing unintended consequences.

On the other hand, Garattini and Walker (Garattini L et al., 2018; Walker A., 2016) say that it is difficult to predict whether the main scores and weights stimulate debate among decision-makers or fortify the role of the technicians who manage the procedure because greater power is given to the people who prepare the scores and weightings. The apparent numerical accuracy of MCDAs can be misleading to decision-makers, giving the false impression that the final results are scientifically proven objective numbers (Garattini L et al. 2018).

Finally, in the EVIDEM framework, which is a multi-stakeholder reflective approach designed to support the culture of reasonable decision-making by promoting procedural and substantive legitimacy, it is proposed that contextual criteria be used as a guide to adapt the frame of reference to the context of decision-making. These criteria may remain in the contextual tool for qualitative considerations by capturing their potential impact qualitatively and thereby affecting the classification or when the framework is adapted to a particular context they may be added to the central MCDA model for quantitative analysis (Wagner M et al., 2016), although its inclusion in the generic additive equation would make the MCDA model spurious because it is the evaluation of these subjective and contextual criteria, while the MCDA model manifests objective technology impacts based on evidence (Radaelli G et al., 2014). Contextual criteria would need a more formal interpretation in the MCDA process since they can sometimes be critical elements for the decision (Walster P et al., 2015). Walster, Goetghebeur and Wagner (Walster P et al., 2015; Goetghebeur MM et al.,

2010; and Wagner M et al., 2017) indicate that MCDA estimates should not be used as a formula approach, but as a guide in decision-making that would allow all relevant quantifiable elements to be unraveled, and then consider the impact of other ethical and contextual elements that influence overall value.

The main limitation of the study is representation at the international level. Clearly, individuals vary in their assessments, which can be influenced by personal and professional factors, such as experience, role in society, and education. This study was not designed to investigate the impact of these criteria on assessments but to make a proposal for their implementation in HTA agency reports; however, it included a diversity of stakeholders (health care consumers, health care providers, managers, academics, etc.) in an attempt to capture a wide variety of perspectives. On the other hand, it facilitates discussions and the exchange of comments, which allowed for a more in-depth analysis of the different aspects involved.

Conclusion

- The selected criteria should be taken into account by HTA agencies when collecting and synthesizing information for pharmacist decision-making.
- The consensus group does not consider that some of the domains should be weighed above others or that individual criteria are more preeminent than others.
- It is proposed to include in the information to be retrieved in the HTA process, all that necessary to respond to deliberative decision-making processes.
- These models can serve as a frame of reference in a systematic and structured discussion based on individual criteria and the evidence supporting them.
- Structured and informed deliberative models can have a certain advantage over closed and uninformed decision-making processes,

as they make explicit and transparent the reasoning behind the final decision.

REFERENCES

Aenishaenslin, C; Gern, L; Michel, P; Ravel, A; Hongoh, V; Waaub, JP; et al. Adaptation and Evaluation of a Multi-Criteria Decision Analysis Model for Lyme Disease Prevention. *PLoS One.*, 2015, 10(8), e0135171.

Angelis, A; Kanavos, P. Multiple Criteria Decision Analysis (MCDA) for evaluating new medicines in Health Technology Assessment and beyond: The Advance Value Framework. *Soc Sci Med.*, 2017 Sep, 188, 137-56.

Annemans, L; Ayme, S; Le Cam, Y; Facey, K; Gunther, P; Nicod, E; et al. Recommendations from the European Working Group for Value Assessment and Funding Processes in Rare Diseases (ORPH-VAL). *Orphanet Journal of Rare Diseases.*, 2017, 12, 50.

Baltussen, R; Stolk, E; Chisholm, D; Aikins, M. Towards a multi-criteria approach for priority setting: an application to Ghana. *Health Econ.*, 2006 Jul, 15(7), 689-96.

Belton, V; Stewart, TJ. *Multiple Criteria Decision Analysis: An integrated Approach*. Kluwer Academic Publishers., 2002.

Brixner, D; Maniadakis, N; Kalo, Z; Hu, S; Shen, J; Wijaya, K. Applying Multi-Criteria Decision Analysis (MCDA) Simple Scoring as an Evidence-based HTA Methodology for Evaluating Off-Patent Pharmaceuticals (OPPs) in Emerging Markets. *Value Health Reg Issues.*, 2017 Sep, 13, 1-6.

Campillo-Artero, C; Puig-Junoy, J; Culyer, AJ. Does MCDA Trump CEA? *Appl Health Econ & Health Pol.*, 2018 Apr, 16(2), 157-61.

Campillo-Artero, C; Puig-Junoy, J. *Rivalry or complementarity between multi-criteria decision analysis and cost-effectiveness analysis?* GCS [Internet]. 2018, 2D(2), 43-45. Available at: http://iiss.es/gcs/ gestion68.pdf.

Castro Jaramillo, HE; Goetghebeur, M; Moreno-Mattar, O. Testing multi-criteria decision analysis for more transparent resource-allocation decision making in Colombia. *Int J Technol Assess Health Care.*, 2016 Jan, 32(4), 307-14.

Cromwell, I; Peacock, SJ; Mitton, C. 'Real-world' health care priority setting using explicit decision criteria: a systematic review of the literature. *BMC Health Serv Res.*, 2015, 15, 164.

Culyer, AJ. Where are the Limits of Cost-Effectiveness Analysis and Health Technology Assessment. *J Med Assoc Thai.*, 2014, 97, (Suppl. 5), S1-S2.

Defechereux, T; Paolucci, F; Mirelman, A; Youngkong, S; Botten, G; Hagen, TP; et al. Health care priority setting in Norway a multicriteria decision analysis. *BMC Health Serv Res.*, 2012, Feb 15, 12, 39.

Dionne, F; Mitton, C; Dempster, B; Lynd, LD. Developing a multi-criteria approach for drug reimbursement decision-making: an initial step forward. *J Popul Ther Clin Pharmacol.*, 2015, 22(1), e68-e77.

Dionne, F; Mitton, C; Macdonald, T; Miller, C; Brennan, M. The challenge of obtaining information necessary for multi-criteria decision analysis implementation: the case of physiotherapy services in Canada. *Cost Eff Resour Alloc.*, 2013, May 20, 11(1), 11.

Drake, JI; de Hart, JCT; Monleon, C; Toro, W; Valentim, J. Utilization of multiple-criteria decision analysis (MCDA) to support healthcare decisionmaking FIFARMA, 2016. *JMark Access Health Policy.*, 2017, 5(1), 1360545.

Frutos Pérez-Surio, A; Gimeno-Gracia, M; Alcácera López, MA; et al. Systematic review for the development of a pharmaceutical and medical products prioritization framework. *J of Pharm Policy and Pract.*, 2019, 12, 21.

Frutos Pérez-Surio, A; Lozano Ortíz, JR. The use of medicines in exceptional circumstances in Spain: adding perspective to early access. *Drugs Ther Perspect*, 2019, 35, 86–92.

Frutos Pérez-Surio, A; Lozano Ortíz, R. Addendum: the use of medicines in exceptional circumstances in Spain: adding perspective to early access. *Drugs Ther Perspect*, 2019, 35, 429–430.

Frutos Pérez-Surio, A; Jordán de Luna, C. *Guidelines for evidence synthesis reporting: medications European Journal of Hospital Pharmacy Published Online First,* 16 November 2018.

Frutos PérezSurio, A; Sala-Piñol, F; Sanmartí-Martinez, N. *Eur J Hosp Pharm,* 2016, 23, 308–313

Garattini, L; Padula, A. Multiple criteria decision analysis in health technology assessment for drugs: Just another illusion? *Appl Health Econ Health Policy.,* 2018, 16(1), 1-4.

Gilabert-Perramon, A; Torrent-Farnell, J; Catalan, A; Prat, A; Fontanet, M; Puig-Peiro, R; et al. Drug evaluation and decision-making in Catalonia: development and validation of a methodological framework based on Multi- criteria decision analysis (MCDA) for orphan drugs. *Int J Technol Assess Health Care.,* 2017 Jan, 33(1), 111-20.

Goetghebeur, MM; Wagner, M; Khoury, H; Rindress, D; Gregoire, JP; Deal, C. Combining multicriteria decision analysis, ethics and health technology assessment: applying the EVIDEM decision-making framework to growth hormone for Turner syndrome patients. *Cost Eff Resour Alloc.,* 2010 Apr 8, 8, 4.

Golan, O; Hansen, P. Which health technologies should be funded? A prioritization framework based explicitly on value for money. *Isr J Health Policy Res.,* 2012 Nov 26, 1(1), 44.

Guindo, LA; Wagner, M; Baltussen, R; Rindress, D; van, TJ; Kind, P; et al. From efficacy to equity: Literature review of decision criteria for resource allocation and healthcare decisionmaking. *Cost Eff Resour Alloc.,* 2012 Jul 18, 10(1), 9.

Holdsworth, M; El, AJ; Bour, A; Kameli, Y; Derouiche, A; Millstone, E; et al. Developing national obesity policy in middle-income countries: a case study from North Africa. *Health Policy Plan.,* 2013 Dec, 28(8), 858-70.

Hongoh, V; Campagna, C; Panic, M; Samuel, O; Gosselin, P; Waaub, JP; et al. Assessing Interventions to Manage West Nile Virus Using Multi-Criteria Decision Analysis with Risk Scenarios. *PLoS One.,* 2016, 11(8), e0160651.

Hoshikawa, K; Ono, S. Discrepancies between multicriteria decision analysis-based ranking and intuitive ranking for pharmaceutical benefit-risk profiles in a hypothetical setting. *J Clin Pharm Ther.*, 2017 Feb, 42(1), 80-86.

Iskrov, G; Miteva-Katrandzhieva, T; Stefanov, R. Multi-Criteria Decision Analysis for Assessment and Appraisal of Orphan Drugs. *Front Public Health*, 2016, 4, 214.

Jehu-Appiah, C; Baltussen, R; Acquah, C; Aikins, M; d'Almeida, SA; Bosu, WK; et al. Balancing equity and efficiency in health priorities in Ghana: the use of multicriteria decision analysis. *Value Health.*, 2008 Dec, 11(7), 1081-7.

Kolasa, K; Zwolinski, KM; Kalo, Z; Hermanowski, T. Potential impact of the implementation of multiple-criteria decision analysis (MCDA) on the Polish pricing and reimbursement process of orphan drugs. *Orphanet J Rare Dis.*, 2016 Mar 10, 11, 23.

Le Gales, C; Moatti, JP. Searching for consensus through multi-criteria decision analysis. Assessment of screening strategies for hemoglobinopathies in southeastern France. *Int J Technol Assess Health Care.*, 1990, 6(3), 430-49.

Marjan Hummel, JM; Snoek, GJ; van Til, JA; Van, RW; IJzerman, MJ. A multicriteria decision analysis of augmentative treatment of upper limbs in persons with tetraplegia. *Journal of Rehabilitation Research and Development.*, 2005 Sep, 42(5), 635-43.

Marsh, K; Ganz, ML; Hsu, J; Strandberg-Larsen, M; Gonzalez, RP; Lund, N. Expanding Health Technology Assessments to Include Effects on the Environment. *Value Health.*, 2016 Mar, 19(2), 249-54.

Marsh, K; Ijzerman, M; Thokala, P; Baltussen, R; Boysen, M; Kalo, Z; et al. Multiple Criteria Decision Analysis for Health Care Decision Making: Emerging good practices: Report 2 of the ISPOR MCDA Emerging Good Practices Task Force. *Value in Health.*, 2016 Mar-Apr, 19(2), 125-137.

Marsh, K; Lanitis, T; Neasham, D; et al. Assessing the value of health care interventions using multi-criteria decision analysis: a review of the literature. *Pharmacoeconomics.*, 2014, 32, 345-365.

Marsh, KD; Sculpher, M; Caro, JJ; Tervonen, T. The Use of MCDA in HTA: Great Potential, but More Effort Needed. *Value Health.*, 2018 Apr, 21(4), 394-397.

Martelli, N; Hansen, P; van den Brink, H; Boudard, A; Cordonnier, AL; Devaux, C; et al. Combining multi-criteria decision analysis and mini-health technology assessment: A funding decision-support tool for medical devices in a university hospital setting. *J Biomed Inform.*, 2016 Feb, 59, 201-8.

Mirelman, A; Mentzakis, E; Kinter, E; Paolucci, F; Fordham, R; Ozawa, S; et al. Decision-making criteria among national policymakers in five countries: a discrete choice experiment eliciting relative preferences for equity and efficiency. *Value Health.*, 2012 May, 15(3), 534-9.

Mobinizadeh, M; Raeissi, P; Nasiripour, AA; Olyaeemanesh, A; Tabibi, SJ. The health systems' priority setting criteria for selecting health technologies: A systematic review of the current evidence. *Med J Islam Repub Iran.*, 2016, 30, 329.

Mohamadi, E; Tabatabaei, SM; Olyaeemanesh, A; Sagha, SF; Zanganeh, M; Davari, M; et al. Coverage decision-making for orthopedics interventions in the health transformation program in Iran: A multiple criteria decision analysis (MCDA). *Shiraz E Medical Journal.*, 2016, 17(12), e40920.

Mullen, PM. Quantifying priorities in healthcare: transparency or illusion? *Health Serv Manage Res.*, 2014, 17, 47-58.

Ottardi, C; Damonti, A; Porazzi, E; Foglia, E; Ferrario, L; Villa, T; et al. A comparative analysis of a disposable and a reusable pedicle screw instrument kit for lumbar arthrodesis: integrating HTA and MCDA. *Health Econ Rev.*, 2017 Dec, 7(1), 17.

Phelps, CE; Madhavan, G. Using Multicriteria Approaches to Assess the Value of Health Care. *Value Health.*, 2017 Feb, 20(2), 251-5.

Poulin, P; Austen, L; Scott, CM; Waddell, CD; Dixon, E; Poulin, M; et al. Multi-criteria development and incorporation into decision tools for health technology adoption. *J Health Organ Manag.*, 2013, 27(2), 246-65.

Radaelli, G; Lettieri, E; Masella, C; Merlino, L; Strada, A; Tringali, M. Implementation of EUnetHTA core Model(®) in Lombardia: the VTS framework. *Int J Technol Assess Health Care.*, 2014 Jan, 30(1), 105-12.

Ritrovato, M; Faggiano, FC; Tedesco, G; Derrico, P. Decision-Oriented Health Technology Assessment: One Step Forward in Supporting the Decision-Making Process in Hospitals. *Value Health.*, 2015 Jun, 18(4), 505-11.

Schmitz, S; McCullagh, L; Adams, R; Barry, M; Walsh, C. Identifying and Revealing the Importance of Decision-Making Criteria for Health Technology Assessment: A Retrospective Analysis of Reimbursement Recommendations in Ireland. *Pharmacoeconomics.*, 2016 Sep, 34(9), 925-37.

Tanios, N; Wagner, M; Tony, M; Baltussen, R; van, TJ; Rindress, D; et al. Which criteria are considered in healthcare decisions? Insights from an international survey of policy and clinical decision makers. *International Journal of Technology Assessment in Health Care.*, 2013 Oct, 29(4), 456-65.

Thokala, P; Devlinb, N; Mars, K; Baltussen, R; Boysen, M; Kalo, Z; et al. Multiple Criteria Decision Analysis for Health Care Decision Making An Introduction: Report 1 of the ISPOR MCDA Emerging Good Practices Task Force. *Value in Health.*, 2016, 19(1), 1-13.

Thokala, P; Duenas, A. Multiple Criteria Decision Analysis for Health Technology Assessment. *Value in health.*, 2012, 5(8), 1172-1181.

Tromp, N; Baltussen, R. Mapping of multiple criteria for priority setting of health interventions: an aid for decision makers. *BMC Health Serv Res.*, 2012 Dec 13, 12, 454.

Venhorst, K; Zelle, SG; Tromp, N; Lauer, JA. Multi-criteria decision analysis of breast cancer control in low- and middle- income countries: development of a rating tool for policy makers. *Cost Eff Resour Alloc.*, 2014, 12, 13.

Wagner, M; Khoury, H; Bennetts, L; Berto, P; Ehreth, J; Badia, X; et al. Appraising the holistic value of Lenvatinib for radio-iodine refractory differentiated thyroid cancer: A multi-country study applying pragmatic MCDA. *BMC Cancer.*, 2017 Apr 17, 17(1), 272.

Wagner, M; Khoury, H; Willet, J; Rindress, D; Goetghebeur, M. Can the EVIDEM Framework Tackle Issues Raised by Evaluating Treatments for Rare Diseases: Analysis of Issues and Policies, and Context-Specific Adaptation. *Pharmacoeconomics.*, 2016 Mar, 34(3), 285-301.

Wahlster, P; Goetghebeur, M; Kriza, C; Niederlander, C; Kolominsky-Rabas, P. Balancing costs and benefits at different stages of medical innovation: a systematic review of Multi-criteria decision analysis (MCDA). *BMC Health Serv Res.*, 2015 Jul 9, 15, 262.

Wahlster, P; Goetghebeur, M; Schaller, S; Kriza, C; Kolominsky-Rabas, P. Exploring the perspectives and preferences for HTA across German healthcare stakeholders using a multi-criteria assessment of a pulmonary heart sensor as a case study. *Health Res Policy Syst.*, 2015, Apr 28, 13, 24.

Walker, A. Challenges in Using MCDA for Reimbursement Decisions on New Medicines? *Value Health.*, 2016 Mar-Apr, 19(2), 123-4.

Youngkong, S; Baltussen, R; Tantivess, S; Mohara, A; Teerawattananon, Y. Multicriteria decision analysis for including health interventions in the universal health coverage benefit package in Thailand. *Value Health.*, 2012 Sep, 15(6), 961-70.

Youngkong, S; Teerawattananon, Y; Tantivess, S; Baltussen, R. Multi-criteria decision analysis for setting priorities on HIV/AIDS interventions in Thailand. *Health Res Policy Syst.*, 2012, Feb 17, 10, 6.

INDEX

A

access, 16, 44, 48, 50, 53, 78, 84, 89, 92, 118, 124, 127, 142, 143, 150, 152, 173, 181
accessibility, 50, 55, 85, 95, 155, 166
alternative medicine, 77, 123
antibiotic, 84, 88, 104, 117, 135, 140, 141, 150, 160
antibiotic resistance, 84, 88, 140
assessment, vii, xi, 10, 20, 41, 47, 75, 76, 78, 92, 93, 95, 97, 98, 100, 108, 114, 124, 125, 127, 128, 151, 152, 154, 163, 164, 165, 166, 173, 176, 182, 184, 186
assessment tools, 76, 97, 125
asthma, 55, 106, 107, 114, 122
awareness, xi, 4, 9, 19, 54, 84, 87, 88, 111, 112, 113, 125, 130, 131, 138, 143, 145, 146, 153, 157

B

barriers, xi, 19, 20, 74, 75, 77, 82, 85, 98, 116, 119, 123, 126, 127, 128, 130, 147, 148, 151, 155

behaviors, 124, 138, 155
benefits, xi, 17, 152, 154, 164, 165, 166, 175, 186
binge eating disorder, 128
birth control, 48
blood, 50, 52, 137, 138, 159
blood pressure, 137, 159

C

campaigns, 87, 90, 147
cancer, ix, 36, 39, 40, 41, 42, 45, 47, 48, 50, 51, 53, 54, 55, 61, 62, 63, 64, 65, 68, 110, 138, 139, 140, 143, 159, 185
cancer therapy, ix, 39, 41
cardiovascular disease, 40, 71, 128, 137, 143
cardiovascular diseases, 40, 137, 143
challenges, v, vii, ix, x, 16, 19, 24, 29, 39, 40, 43, 45, 48, 53, 54, 55, 69, 70, 73, 75, 77, 79, 81, 82, 88, 90, 91, 92, 96, 98, 105, 108, 112, 113, 117, 123, 127, 129, 147, 148, 151, 157, 162, 186
chemotherapeutic agent, 40, 42, 43, 45, 139
chemotherapy, vii, ix, 37, 39, 41, 42, 43, 44, 45, 46, 48, 49, 52, 53, 64, 66, 110

chronic diseases, 40, 55, 71, 86, 89, 128, 130, 131, 138, 144, 147
chronic illness, 118, 143, 149, 153
chronic obstructive pulmonary disease, 107
clinical examination, 126, 127
clinical oncology, 62, 68
clinical pharmacy, x, 4, 5, 6, 12, 13, 14, 15, 30, 41, 64, 65, 95, 97, 130, 131, 135, 138, 141, 144, 145, 146, 151, 156
colon cancer, 66
colorectal cancer, 54, 62, 64, 68
common symptoms, 138
community, viii, x, 2, 9, 10, 11, 14, 16, 36, 70, 72, 76, 81, 82, 84, 85, 90, 91, 93, 95, 96, 97, 102, 104, 105, 106, 108, 111, 113, 115, 116, 119, 122, 124, 125, 127, 128, 130, 131, 133, 134, 136, 138, 140, 141, 142, 143, 145, 146, 147, 149, 150, 151, 152, 153, 155, 156, 158, 159, 160, 161
community pharmacy, x, 9, 11, 76, 102, 115, 116, 122, 125, 130, 131, 133, 142, 143, 146, 153, 161
curricula, 15, 74, 77, 106
curriculum, viii, ix, 2, 12, 15, 17, 24, 25, 26, 30, 31, 77, 79, 101, 108, 111, 132, 152

D

deaths, 40, 45, 134
depression, 82, 90, 139
diabetes, 51, 55, 71, 99, 116, 122, 137, 138, 143, 158, 159
diabetic patients, 35, 36, 101
diastolic blood pressure, 138
diseases, xi, 40, 47, 48, 51, 53, 54, 55, 71, 78, 81, 85, 86, 89, 95, 100, 106, 118, 121, 124, 128, 130, 131, 136, 137, 138, 140, 143, 144, 147, 150, 155, 161
disorder, 112, 128, 173
dosage, 8, 44, 49, 104, 135, 141, 150

dosing, 141, 152
drug addiction, 139
drug delivery, 13, 94
drug interaction, 48, 49, 51, 64, 105, 134, 135, 136, 140, 144, 145, 152, 157
drug reactions, 49, 52, 103, 134, 140, 144, 152, 157
drug therapy, 6, 9, 10, 41, 42, 49, 142
drugs, vii, ix, xi, 5, 6, 35, 39, 40, 42, 43, 44, 45, 46, 51, 53, 87, 89, 95, 106, 107, 130, 131, 133, 135, 138, 139, 140, 141, 144, 147, 149, 150, 151, 153, 157, 171, 182, 183

E

economics, 80, 98, 112
education, v, vii, viii, ix, x, 1, 2, 9, 10, 11, 12, 13, 14, 15, 16, 17, 18, 19, 21, 22, 23, 24, 25, 26, 27, 28, 29, 30, 31, 32, 33, 34, 35, 37, 41, 43, 46, 47, 53, 54, 58, 61, 62, 64, 65, 68, 70, 72, 73, 74, 76, 77, 78, 79, 86, 91, 92, 95, 98, 100, 104, 109, 111, 112, 113, 118, 122, 124, 128, 131, 132, 138, 148, 151, 152, 154, 155, 156, 162, 179
educational experience, 17, 25
educational institutions, x, 14, 18, 70, 74, 92
educational programs, 95, 103
elderly population, 144
emergency, 22, 142
evidence, x, xii, 3, 4, 6, 20, 64, 77, 78, 94, 103, 110, 122, 130, 133, 136, 164, 165, 167, 169, 171, 177, 178, 179, 182, 184
exclusion, xii, 164, 166, 168, 169, 170, 171, 173, 176

F

families, 5, 24
family members, 153

financial, x, 9, 11, 18, 25, 43, 70, 76, 81, 83, 98, 149, 150
financial resources, 9, 18
financial support, 76
funding, 20, 82, 148, 184

G

generic drugs, 87
glucose, 50, 52, 137, 138
governance, x, 70, 88, 91, 151, 162
governments, 154, 156
graduate education, 74
graduate program, 13
growth, 3, 64, 71, 73, 131, 140, 182
growth hormone, 182
guidelines, 37, 43, 51, 92, 93, 108, 115, 139, 160, 174

H

health care, vii, viii, ix, 1, 2, 4, 6, 9, 14, 17, 43, 86, 88, 89, 96, 97, 99, 102, 116, 125, 133, 134, 141, 142, 143, 144, 147, 150, 155, 156, 157, 160, 170, 179, 181, 183
health care professionals, 9, 88, 97, 157
health care system, 147, 155, 156
health information, 142, 143, 173
health services, 10, 82, 130, 153, 165
health status, 6, 173
health technology assessment, vii, xi, 100, 164, 165, 166, 176, 182, 184
heart disease, 55
heart failure, 36, 137
hematology, 6, 35
herbal medicine, 3
HIV, 147, 171, 186
human, xi, 24, 43, 130, 174
hypertension, 51, 55, 131, 137, 138

I

immigrants, 72, 173
immunization, 147, 155
industrial revolution, 131
industry, xi, 3, 10, 73, 97, 164, 166
infection, 9, 141, 160
influenza, 107
insomnia, 82, 114, 139
institutions, viii, x, 1, 5, 11, 14, 17, 18, 19, 26, 47, 55, 70, 74, 79, 80, 91, 92, 97, 154
integration, viii, 2, 15, 24, 25, 28, 49, 92, 146, 161
intensive care unit, 123, 135
international standards, 93, 151, 154
Interprofessional education, x, 2, 17, 70, 111, 113, 151
intervention, 7, 86, 89, 106, 138, 157, 159, 176, 177
irritable bowel syndrome, 36
issues, 9, 42, 43, 44, 54, 71, 78, 83, 86, 88, 98, 134, 143, 144, 145, 151

J

job characteristics, 120
job satisfaction, 82, 102, 120

K

kidney, 52, 110
knowledge acquisition, 20

L

labor market, 74, 75
laws, 147, 151, 155, 156
leadership, 10, 26, 44, 77, 137

learning, vii, viii, x, 1, 2, 9, 14, 15, 16, 17, 18, 19, 20, 21, 22, 24, 25, 70, 74, 75, 78, 96, 106, 108, 122, 127, 146
learning environment, 21, 127
learning outcomes, x, 70, 74
learning process, 21
literacy, 78, 83, 94, 96, 98, 118, 128
loss of appetite, 139
low- and middle-income countries, 82, 130, 132, 162

M

manufacturing, 3, 14, 94, 130, 131, 132, 175
medical, vii, xi, 5, 6, 8, 16, 19, 23, 24, 25, 42, 43, 44, 48, 51, 53, 78, 95, 130, 131, 133, 140, 141, 142, 144, 145, 146, 149, 151, 153, 154, 155, 164, 165, 166, 171, 181, 184, 186
medical history, 24, 53, 146
medical science, 78, 133
medication, ix, x, xi, 3, 4, 5, 7, 8, 9, 19, 25, 27, 40, 43, 45, 46, 48, 50, 53, 70, 80, 81, 82, 83, 84, 85, 86, 88, 94, 95, 96, 97, 99, 100, 101, 102, 104, 106, 110, 115, 116, 117, 118, 121, 122, 123, 126, 130, 131, 132, 134, 135, 136, 138, 140, 142, 143, 144, 145,146, 147, 148, 149, 152, 153, 155, 157
medicine, 3, 4, 6, 8, 12, 14, 16, 44, 77, 78, 95, 99, 110, 117, 122, 123, 125, 137, 147, 153, 158
mental health, 82, 147
Middle East, v, vii, ix, 13, 30, 69, 70, 71, 72, 73, 75, 77, 78, 79, 80, 81, 82, 83, 84, 85, 86, 87, 88, 89, 91, 93, 97, 98, 102, 104, 106, 108, 110, 111, 113, 116, 117, 118, 119, 122, 126, 127
misuse, 84, 85, 88, 97, 104, 117
motivation, 21, 78, 82
multicriteria decision analysis, 165, 181, 182, 183, 186

N

nausea, 37, 51
neurotoxicity, 51
nurses, ix, 8, 40, 46, 49, 95, 115, 139, 141, 145
nursing, 16, 46, 170
nutrition, 6, 147
nutritional status, 90

O

obesity, 71, 171, 182
obstacles, viii, 2, 17, 18, 20, 26, 28, 75
oncology pharmacists, vii, ix, 39, 40, 43, 44, 47, 55
online learning, 24
opportunities, 11, 14, 15, 20, 75, 91, 96, 98, 105, 117, 137, 142, 144, 147, 151
organ(s), 6, 11, 40, 43
outpatient, 45, 95, 100
oversight, 82, 110, 139

P

pain, 6, 130, 139, 140, 159
pain management, 6
participants, 20, 22, 142, 153
patient care, viii, 2, 5, 6, 8, 9, 11, 14, 16, 17, 18, 19, 20, 41, 131, 132, 146, 149, 151
patient outcomes, 19, 85, 94, 130, 131, 132, 135, 138, 141, 142, 145, 152, 161
patient-oriented service, ix, 40
perspectives, v, vii, ix, x, xi, 5, 27, 29, 39, 40, 58, 69, 70, 91, 104, 105, 109, 111, 115, 116, 126, 128, 129, 141, 157, 158, 161, 164, 166, 177, 179, 186

pharmaceutical care, vii, ix, xi, 4, 6, 7, 8, 36, 39, 40, 41, 42, 47, 48, 50, 51, 53, 54, 55, 61, 62, 66, 68, 72, 78, 83, 85, 99, 119, 130, 131, 133, 136, 137, 138, 139, 141, 144, 148, 156, 158, 159
pharmaceutical(s), vii, ix, x, xi, 3, 4, 5, 6, 7, 8, 10, 11, 12, 23, 26, 29, 36, 39, 40, 41, 42, 47, 48, 50, 51, 53, 54, 55, 61, 62, 66, 68, 70, 72, 73, 78, 79, 83, 85, 90, 91, 97, 98, 99, 107, 108, 109, 116, 119, 120, 123, 130, 131, 133, 136, 137, 138, 139, 141, 143, 144, 148,150, 156, 158, 159, 165, 181, 183
pharmacogenetics, 103
pharmacokinetics, 77, 118
pharmacology, 25
pharmacotherapy, 4, 22, 131, 132, 133, 136, 139, 165
pharmacy education, vii, ix, x, 1, 2, 11, 12, 13, 14, 16, 26, 70, 72, 74, 76, 91, 104, 109, 118, 155
physical activity, 90, 138
physicians, 83, 87, 89, 94, 95, 102, 104, 106, 133, 135, 136, 139, 141, 142, 144, 145, 146, 148, 153
population, ix, 11, 70, 71, 72, 87, 89, 90, 92, 98, 110, 113, 114, 118, 123, 128, 133, 144, 150, 154, 169
poverty, 71, 147, 156, 173
practice, v, vii, viii, ix, x, 1, 2, 3, 4, 5, 6, 7, 8, 9, 10, 12, 13, 14, 15, 17, 18, 19, 20, 24, 25, 27, 28, 29, 30, 31, 32, 33, 34, 41, 42, 56, 57, 58, 59, 60, 64, 67, 70, 72, 73, 74, 75, 78, 80, 81, 82, 83, 90, 91, 92, 93, 94, 98, 99, 100, 101, 103, 104, 106, 108, 109, 111, 112, 114, 115, 117, 118, 122, 123, 125, 126, 127, 128, 130, 135, 138, 140, 141, 142, 146, 147, 148, 149, 150, 151, 155, 156, 158, 161, 162, 167, 176
pregnancy, 36, 103, 123
prevention, xi, 5, 41, 50, 52, 96, 97, 107, 110, 130, 147, 155, 175

public health, 71, 86, 100, 118, 127, 143, 147, 149, 150, 155, 162, 165, 171

Q

quality assurance, 9, 73
quality of life, 37, 41, 47, 51, 66, 85, 114, 123, 133, 139, 153
quality of service, 154
quality standards, x, 70, 73, 92, 93

R

radiotherapy, 41, 50
reactions, 23, 49, 52, 95, 103, 134, 135, 136, 140, 144, 152, 157
refugees, 71, 88, 101, 102
regulations, 84, 85, 174
regulatory agencies, 46, 151
research, viii, ix, x, 1, 2, 10, 12, 14, 15, 18, 28, 29, 30, 32, 33, 34, 35, 37, 55, 56, 59, 61, 62, 64, 68, 70, 73, 79, 80, 81, 91, 92, 96, 98, 109, 112, 115, 118, 119, 120, 121, 122, 126, 128, 129, 131, 151, 157, 158, 160, 161, 162, 167, 171, 183
researchers, xii, 80, 87, 97, 98, 135, 154, 164, 170, 173
resistance, 75, 84, 88, 140, 150, 160
resources, xi, 6, 8, 9, 17, 18, 28, 34, 44, 71, 77, 78, 88, 97, 130, 144, 174
risk assessment, 114, 128
risk factors, 36, 110, 114, 116, 121, 135
risk(s), 11, 36, 43, 83, 92, 110, 114, 116, 121, 123, 128, 134, 135, 136, 144, 155, 173, 175, 176, 183

S

safety, 22, 43, 44, 54, 55, 82, 88, 94, 95, 102, 103, 106, 113, 114, 126, 133, 134, 135, 140, 145, 152, 153, 166
school, viii, 2, 9, 12, 14, 16, 17, 23, 128, 155
science, 5, 18, 24, 25, 28, 41, 104, 133
services, x, xi, 4, 6, 7, 9, 10, 12, 13, 16, 19, 21, 41, 47, 50, 55, 64, 70, 72, 81, 82, 84, 85, 88, 90, 95, 96, 97, 102, 103, 107, 128, 130, 132, 133, 134, 143, 146, 147, 149, 151, 152, 153, 154, 155, 159, 161, 165, 181
shortage, 89, 98, 142, 147, 150, 156
side effects, 47, 49, 51, 52, 53, 64, 131, 134, 136, 144, 153
smoking cessation, 93, 155
socioeconomic status, 83, 175
stereotypes, 77, 148
stress, 71, 81, 82, 91, 102, 150
structure, 20, 35, 82, 97, 169
substance abuse, 116
substitution, 77, 87, 105, 106, 111, 124
symptoms, 36, 41, 136, 138
syndrome, 36, 52, 171, 182

T

technologies, ix, xi, xii, 2, 21, 163, 164, 165, 166, 168, 169, 171, 175, 176, 182, 184
technology, vii, xi, 20, 21, 23, 24, 43, 78, 96, 100, 109, 164, 165, 166, 170, 173, 174, 175, 176, 178, 182, 184
therapeutic goal, 41, 47, 50
therapy, ix, 4, 5, 6, 7, 9, 10, 27, 39, 40, 41, 42, 49, 53, 82, 89, 96, 97, 99, 110, 125, 137, 140, 142, 143, 152, 153
tobacco, 86, 112, 147
toxicity, 6, 43, 52, 53
training, vii, viii, 1, 2, 10, 11, 12, 13, 14, 16, 17, 18, 19, 22, 23, 30, 42, 47, 51, 73, 74, 76, 90, 94, 127, 134, 135, 139, 140, 143, 148, 149, 151, 154, 155, 157, 173, 174
training programs, 12, 16, 42, 47, 139
transparency, 91, 98, 108, 184
treatment, ix, xi, 6, 8, 23, 37, 39, 40, 41, 42, 44, 47, 48, 50, 51, 52, 53, 54, 55, 62, 65, 68, 84, 89, 98, 102, 112, 115, 124, 130, 131, 134, 135, 136, 137, 138, 139, 141, 142, 143, 144, 153, 158, 173, 175, 183
trial, 112, 158, 159, 177

U

ulcerative colitis, 36
undergraduate education, 47
universities, 26, 73, 74, 75, 76, 79, 151, 154

V

vaccine, 95, 99, 113
validation, 24, 123, 182
vertical dimensions, 25
vertical integration, 25
vitamin D deficiency, 36
vitamins, 36, 48

W

waste, 43, 90, 154, 175
waste management, 43, 90
well-being, 6, 91, 92
workforce, ix, 2, 90, 91, 105, 109, 114, 161
World Health Organization (WHO), 5, 17, 26, 33, 34, 71, 72, 100, 122, 138, 142, 147, 150, 151, 156, 160
worldwide, 16, 26, 40, 41, 78, 81, 134, 142